PROFESSIONALISM
IN THE PRACTICE
OF PHYSICAL THERAPY

PROFESSIONALISM IN THE PRACTICE OF PHYSICAL THERAPY
A Case-Based Approach

Tonya Y. Miller PT, DPT, PhD
Doctor of Physical Therapy Program Lead
Associate Professor
Harrisburg University of Science and Technology
Harrisburg, Pennsylvania

Laurie Brogan, PT, DPT
Board Certified Geriatric Specialist
Certified Exercise Expert for the Aging Adult
Assistant Professor-Physical Therapy Department
Misericordia University
Dallas, Pennsylvania

McGraw Hill

1 2 3 4 5 6 7 8 9   DSS   29 28 27 26 25 24

ISBN 978-1-264-27863-3
MHID 1-264-27863-2

This book was set in Minion Pro by MPS Limited.
The editors were Michael Weitz and Peter J. Boyle.
The production supervisor was Catherine H. Saggese.
Project management was provided by Poonam Bisht, MPS Limited.

Cataloging-in-publication data for this book is on file at the Library of Congress.

McGraw-Hill books are available at special quantity discounts to use as premiums and sales promotions, or for use in corporate training programs. To contact a representative, please visit the Contact Us pages at www.mhprofessional.com.

Contents

About the Authors

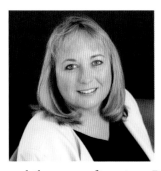

Tonya Y. Miller, PT, DPT, PhD, is the doctor of physical therapy program lead at Harrisburg University of Science and Technology and owner of TYM Coaching, a health care leadership consulting firm. A well-regarded health care leader and national speaker with broad experience in leading teams in both the health care and the nonprofit sectors, Dr. Miller's writing combines over 30 years of real-world clinical leadership with her academic expertise in leadership studies. She is passionate about mentoring and guiding health care professionals through her commitment to integrity, accountability, and self-awareness. Tonya applies these concepts and more in the professional development model throughout her first book, *Professionalism in the Practice of Physical Therapy: A Case-based Approach.*

Tonya resides in Camp Hill, Pennsylvania, with her spouse, Karen Palmer, two dogs, and Sam the Cat. She believes in social responsibility and is an active community and professional organization volunteer. Tonya serves on both local- and national-level boards, including the American Physical Therapy Association, Cumberland & Perry County Domestic Violence Shelter, and PA Vent Camp, a camp for ventilator-dependent children, in which she is the executive director.

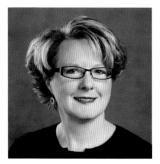

Laurie Brogan, PT, DPT, is a full-time faculty member of the physical therapy department at Misericordia University, primarily responsible for teaching cardiopulmonary physical therapy, clinical skills, and professional development. With strong interests in the needs of the older adult population and interprofessional education/practice, she is also an American Board of Physical Therapy Specialists (ABPTS) Board-Certified Clinical Specialist in Geriatric Physical Therapy, a Certified Exercise Expert for the Aging Adult, and a Certified Master Trainer for TeamSTEPPS, a program developed by the Agency for Healthcare Research and Quality (AHRQ) and the Department of Defense as a solution to improving collaboration and communication in health care settings. Her research and writing centers around interprofessional education and practice, socialization in interprofessional settings, and the development of clinical reasoning in PT education. She is committed to providing quality physical therapy education.

Laurie resides in Pittston, Pennsylvania, with her spouse, Michael. She is active in the American Physical Therapy Association's regional, state, and national sectors and is dedicated to serving others through engagement in various community service organizations.

Foreword

Exploration of professionalism within physical therapy is a multifaceted concept examined by the authors of this book. Drawing from extensive experience and a dedication to individualized growth and development, the authors have crafted an accessible exploration of this subject. The narrative embarks on an engaging journey, unveiling layers of insights through succinct and purposeful chapters enriched with models, case studies, and contemplative reflections.

Within these pages, the authors interweave the threads of individual, professional, and societal responsibilities, inviting every reader, regardless of their experience in the profession, to embark on a personal journey of discovery. Readers are encouraged to engage in introspection, reflect on their personal encounters, and gain valuable insights into their interactions with others. Each chapter provides information and perspective, fostering an environment where readers can identify, build upon, and confront their knowledge, experiences, and challenges.

Structured as stepping stones, the chapters serve as a pathway for readers to identify and navigate their professional journey. The aim is to empower physical therapy professionals to chart a purposeful course using this text as a compass for personal and career development in their community.

Roger Herr, PT, MPA
Vice President, VNS Health
APTA Board President 2021-2024

Preface

As the world of health care continues to evolve and change, so does the idea of professionalism. No longer is it noted simply by title, role, or education. In today's interconnected and global society, the importance of professional behavior and the cultivation of a solid commitment to personal development are paramount to any health care practitioner's ultimate personal and professional success. The health care environment is a mosaic of diversity, with professionals from various backgrounds, cultures, and experiences coming together to meet the needs of an equally diverse workforce and patient population.

One cannot overstate the importance of professionalism and the continuous pursuit of personal development through lifelong learning. The significance of growth extends beyond the practitioner to the clients we serve and the health care community in which we work. True professionals are not static entities. A commitment to growth does not solely benefit one's career but can have ripple effects that profoundly influence those around us. Professionalism becomes the glue that fosters collaboration, trust, and improved outcomes.

Physical therapy requires many talents, including knowledge, clinical expertise, and compassion. The integration of these traits relies heavily on professionalism—a concept that encompasses such attributes as effective communication, cultural competence, social responsibility, ethical conduct, and a commitment to lifelong learning. These attributes build on the foundation of emotional intelligence, grit, and resilience. These traits are desirable and necessary for every physical therapy practitioner, regardless of their years of experience. It is never too late for self-improvement!

Welcome to *Professionalism in the Practice of Physical Therapy: A Case-based Approach*. In designing this textbook, we intended it to serve the student, educator, and practicing physical therapists and physical therapists' assistants. The book's design provides thought, discussion, and direction for professional development. We grounded the book in current knowledge and theory but designed it as a dynamic tool to engage the learner in real-world scenarios and practical challenges through case studies. These case studies allow one to examine the complexity of modern-day professionalism within physical therapy and throughout the health care continuum. It directs one toward the creation of a professional development plan that is flexible. The flexible plan allows for modification as you navigate contemporary health care throughout your career.

The authors share a passion for this topic. With many years of working in health care and teaching, this book is a culmination of many discussions and a shared strong belief that self-discovery and awareness of the world around is a catalyst for growth. It is our hope that you use these case studies, the accompanying reflection questions, and the professional development plan to stimulate thought and discussion that enhance your awareness and understanding of professionalism and help you find inspiration and insight into your own journey of personal and professional growth.

pro·fes·sion·al·ism

the conduct, aims, or qualities that characterize
or mark a profession or a professional person

Merriam-Webster.com Dictionary

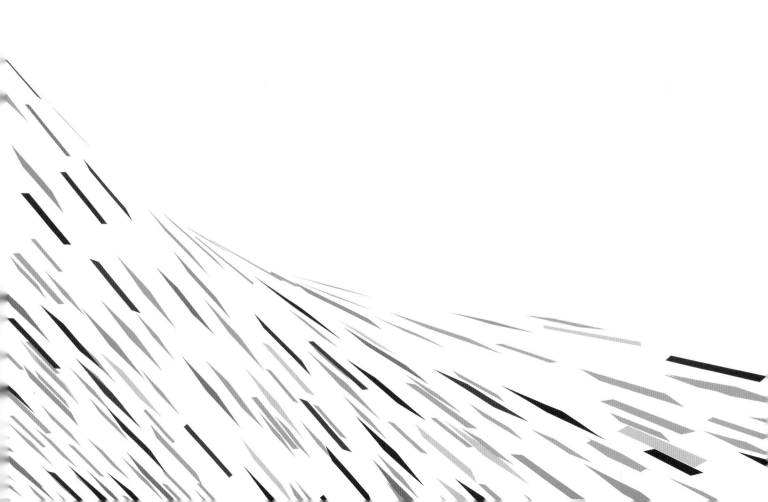

chapter 1

Introduction to Professionalism

● HOW TO USE THIS BOOK

Though hard to describe, professionalism is an essential tenet of most health care professions. It is vital for those working in professions to build relationships that require awareness of self and others. Professionalism is a concept that impacts students and the educational experience as well as practitioners within all practice settings. Professionalism can impact the overall image of self and others. The purpose of this book is to facilitate professional growth for both students and experienced clinicians. Its concepts apply to students, early careerists, and those seeking to examine the professional realm within physical therapy. It fits nicely into an educational term/semester by supporting creation of personal development plan. This book facilitates introspection and discussion by highlighting the challenges and opportunities within the realm of professionalism and professional growth.

This book is presented in three parts. The design of the first part allows the reader to gain a basic overview of professionalism in health care from a historical perspective with future considerations. It offers an overview of the potential definitions and measures of professionalism and seeks to define some levels of professional growth that occur with awareness and a strategic development plan. Before starting the second part of this book, the reader should take some time to reflect on their overall current thoughts on professionalism based on the general concepts discussed in Part 1.

In Part 2 of this book, the reader explores concepts of professionalism through element descriptions, case studies, and personal reflection. This part of the book provides stimulation for discussion and personal growth. Each chapter guides the reader through a key tenet of professionalism that culminates in a case study that allows an opportunity to determine one's current professional position related to the scenario. These case studies are examples of how physical therapists may respond to the situation and allow an opportunity to reflect and set development goals by utilizing a three-level hierarchy of professionalism. The

three levels of professionalism are the emerging professional, the reflective professional, and the influencing professional. These three levels utilize the symbolism of the oak tree as a sign of growth throughout one's career.

Finally, Part 3 of this book guides the reader through a professional strategic development plan. In this part, the reader explores how mentorship, personal goal-setting, and lifelong reflection contribute to professional growth. By working through this book, the reader develops a foundational knowledge of professionalism, gains insight into professional development, and learns strategies necessary to grow professionally throughout their career. Although the focus audience for this book is students and entry-level careerists, its contents apply across the continuum of a physical therapist's career. Returning to this book throughout one's career allows the reader to reexamine professional growth and establish new goals to ensure continued personal and professional development.

● DEFINING PROFESSIONALISM IN HEALTH CARE – A CONUNDRUM

At first thought, it may seem easy to describe professionalism. The professional is commonly used to describe individuals from different walks of life and roles. If we pause for a second, each of us could produce an image of a professional in our minds. Maybe the image of a physician, a computer analyst, or an engineer appears. We easily label these individuals as professionals, but why? What specific attributes mark these individuals as professionals? Is it their education, their level of authority, a common trait they all share, or maybe the work environment or their social role? They all certainly have different roles and different levels of education. So maybe it's the common traits? If so, what are those traits, and why do those specific traits matter? Therein lies the conundrum of describing professionalism. Like so many other tangibles, professionalism has meant different things to different groups of people throughout history. The fact of the matter is that professionalism is not a static concept. Professionalism is an evolving dynamic construct that is often challenging to define, let alone assess. It is worth taking a step back and examining a brief history of professionalism in health care, particularly the physical therapy profession, the current literature supporting some of today's constructs of health care professionalism, and where the future may lead us.

● HISTORY OF PROFESSIONALISM IN MEDICINE

Professionalism in Ancient Times

Looking back, we find examples of professionalism throughout the healing practices. Eastern and Western cultures describe the need for a certain level of a calling or conduct from those considered healers. We can trace the origins of healers back to ancient times. For example, in the ancient text *Charaka Samhita* (400 BC), considered the first text of Ayurvedic medicine, an ancient Indian holistic healing practice, references exist to the importance of the healer's code of conduct. The *Charaka Samhita* states that those who practice because of compassion for living beings and not for money or caprice are the best among the healers. Likewise, Hippocrates (460-377 BC), considered the father of Western medicine, wrote the Hippocratic Oath based on the premise of doing no harm and understanding that the healer held a level of power and should not use that power for personal gain. Additionally, a Chinese medical ethicist Sun Simiao (1200-1300 AD) wrote that physicians should treat all humans equally regardless of status, wealth, age, friend or enemy, or even personal attractiveness. These early examples not only guide today's ideas of professionalism, but also demonstrate the need for individuals in the healing practice to understand their responsibilities to others.[1,2]

A Renaissance of Professionalism

Although little was done to move the healing professions forward in the Middle Ages, healers of the Renaissance era took a renewed interest in the conduct and ethics of the healing practitioner. One of the earliest expressions of medical ethics conduct, the Hippocratic Oath remained a guiding principle where practitioners pledged their individual code of moral conduct. To this point in history, the codes of conduct focused solely on the responsibility of each individual practitioner.[1]

The idea of a group of individuals sharing common values and code of conduct, thus defining a profession, did not evolve until more recently. In 1803, following a breakdown in medical care during a typhoid epidemic, Thomas Percival, an English surgeon, authored a book entitled *Medical Ethics, or a Code of Institutes and Precepts, Adapted to the Professional Conduct of Physicians and Surgeons*. This book established the foundational thinking of professionalism as something beyond the individual responsibility but as a collective responsibility of the collective group or "the profession." In this book, Percival outlines professional duty as a unified responsibility to care for the sick. The ideas from Percival's book spread throughout the world. In the United States, it became the guiding document for the American Medical Association (AMA) Code of Medical Ethics in 1847.[1]

Although the foundation of the AMA Code of Medical Ethics provided core principles of professional duty, the profession of medicine still had a long journey toward our current views on professionalism. Throughout the early and mid-1900s, medicine continued to evolve and debate the concepts of professionalism and its relationship to the role of health care providers.

Modern-Day Professionalism

Several developments occurred throughout the last century, which further evolved into our current construct of health care as a profession. In the early 1900s, medicine and medical schools, especially in the United States, were largely unregulated and varied greatly in standards of conduct. A 1910 report by Abraham Flexner, known as the Flexner Report, brought to light the challenges facing medicine and the education of those practicing medicine. The Flexner Report greatly influenced medical education standards, thus elevating medical practitioners' conduct level.

Other events continued to shape our current thinking about the meaning of professionalism in medicine. In the 1960s and 1970s, medicine and medical education again came under public scrutiny. In this new era of consumerism, the public began questioning the authority of medicine and the collective motives of those practicing medicine. This scrutiny led to the creation of patient-focused concepts guiding the acceptable conduct of the medical profession. In the 1970s, a field of study known as bioethics emerged from this debate. Unlike medical ethics, which focuses on the medical profession's duty, bioethics focuses on patients' rights. Bioethics profoundly impacted the role of medicine in society. It questioned the altruism of medicine toward the patient, extending beyond the measure of medical outcomes. The continued debate between medical ethicists and bioethicists through the late 1900s further defined the collective conduct of those practicing medicine.

The debate of the late 1900s led the American Board of Internal Medicine (ABIM) to establish "Project Professionalism" with the following goals: (1) define professionalism, (2) raise the concept of professionalism in the consciousness of all within internal medicine, (3) provide a means for program directors to inculcate the concepts of professionalism within their training programs, and (4) develop strategies for assessing the professionalism of residents and subspecialty fellows during training.[3] This document established an educational framework for professionalism in medical schools. The ABIM later developed the Physician Charter in 2002 to further clarify its commitment to professionalism. The Physician Charter is a statement of fundamental principles of medical professionalism. The fundamental principles held three key values: (1) altruism, (2) patient autonomy, and (3) social justice. The Physician Charter became a guiding document not only for physician practice in the 21st century but also a guiding document for other health care professions, such as physical therapy.[1,3–5]

As this historical context demonstrates, professionalism is a complex concept. Historically, we see that professionalism evolved from the individual responsibilities of professionalism through the 18th century to examining what professionalism means to a collective group of individuals. The discourse of professionalism as individual traits or attributes and factors impacting groups or societies continues today. When examining professionalism in day-to-day interactions, it is important to have a framework for discussion.

Professionalism in the 21st Century

In 2010, the International Ottawa Conference Working Group on the Assessment of Professionalism was created. This research group consisted of medical and health care professional educators from nine countries representing a variety of clinical practice and academic disciplines. This group used discourse analysis to identify and define elements and assess professionalism. They viewed professionalism through individual, interpersonal, and societal/institutional realms and then developed eight guiding principles for assessing professionalism. These guiding principles, summarized in **Table 1.1** below, help shape how we consider professionalism in the 21st century.[6]

Those familiar with the core documents that guide the current practice of physical therapy will recognize how the perspective of medicine and the concepts of individual, interpersonal, and societal-institutional impact have influenced professionalism within our field. In Part 2 of this book, we present case studies examining components of professionalism. Through these case studies, we discuss the scenarios through the individual, interpersonal, or societal lens. Referring back to this part as a framework for those discussions may be helpful.

Individual – Attributes, Character, Attitudes, Behaviors, and Identities – The individual lens considers personal moral drivers and attributes within the person. There are two approaches to the individual lens. The first approach examines the individual level from the perspective that many of these attributes are

TABLE 1.1.   Ottawa Conference Working Group Guiding Principles
Principle 1: Professionalism varies throughout history and across cultures.
Principle 2: There is an ongoing need to develop a more concrete definition and defensible assessment across medical educators.
Principle 3: Professionalism is fluid and reflective of societal and health care changes. Requires periodic redefinition.
Principle 4: Medical educators must engage society in ongoing dialogue to gain a comprehensive understanding of professionalism.
Principle 5: Measurement of levels of professionalism requires both summative and formative evaluation recognizing the value of feedback and remediation along the lifespan of students and practitioners.
Principle 6: Historically, supporting literature of professionalism arose from Anglo-Saxon countries. One must proceed with caution when transferring these ideas to other contexts and cultures.
Principle 7: Diversity of approaches and perspectives must be incorporated into the education, assessment, and research of professionalism.
Principle 8: Perspectives will impact attention to varying elements of professionalism. The framework of the individual elements of professionalism is vast and may, at times, conflict.

Adapted from "Assessment of Professionalism: Recommendations from the Ottawa 2010 Conference," Hodges BD, Ginsburg S, Cruess R. Med Teach. 2011;33(5):354-363. doi:10.3109/0142159X.2011.577300.

innate to the person and strengthen over time. The other perspective examines the individual from a development model in which one obtains these attributes and gains insight into application over the course of education and mentoring. Both views provide value to the perspective of how individuals develop their own traits and attributes of professionalism.[6]

Although examining professionalism through the individual lens seems reasonable, this perspective has many challenges. First, the literature has yet to agree on which traits and characteristics best predict future behaviors. Second, using specific traits and characteristics to measure one's future ability to effectively perform a set of behaviors or fulfill a societal role may limit some from future roles and responsibilities. This is especially true when considering the individual lens from the development model, in which attributes and traits evolve over the course of time and through specific actions.

Interpersonal – Relationships, Group Dynamics, Cultural Consideration, and Context – This lens focuses on the context of the interactions between individuals, therefore creating a more fluid concept of professionalism. Assessing professionalism through this lens allows the individuals to co-create the aspects of professionalism based on the current environment and engagement of the two individuals. This lens is contextually driven. Consider those whom you interact with in a variety of settings. The attributes and traits necessary to interact with others in different environments vary based on the context of that setting. For example, interactions with community members vary based on the setting. An interaction at the local hospital may differ greatly from one at the local gym or grocery store. Is that medical professional any less of a professional in a casual setting or a more formal setting? This lens allows the context of the environment and situation to drive the interaction and shape the response.[6]

From the perspective of the interpersonal lens, "Professionalism is considered a set of socio-cognitive processes that individuals use to interpret the world and to select appropriate responses in relation to others."[6] The concepts of specific traits or characteristics being professional or unprofessional become less important through this lens. Rather, an individual is seen as having a professionalism lapse when not interpreting or responding to a situation according to the level of behavior necessary for the context of the situation.[6]

A challenge with the interpersonal lens is that one must integrate the contextual aspects of the situation, including all individuals in the interaction within the physical environment, to assess professionalism fully. Integrating this complex system to understand professionalism presents challenges in resources and replication of assessment.

Societal/Institutional – Economic, Political, Organizational, Civil – Through this lens, professionalism is defined with and by society. Society constructs the role of the professional group and the state of being professional. Professions serve a societal function and a specific expectation and power level based on the profession's role. The role of the individual and interpersonal lens are components of the overall societal construct and expectations of the collective group or the profession. In this lens, a measure of the professional or profession comes from macro, or societal, impacts such as patient outcomes or acceptable adherence to standards such as accreditation.[6] The collective core values or approaches tied to a specific philosophy arise from the societal/institutional lens of assessing professionalism. Thus, the societal lens demonstrates its usefulness in establishing normative behaviors of groups within society.[6]

Like the individual and interpersonal lenses, challenges in applying the societal/institutional viewpoint to assessing professionalism exist. For example, because the societal/institutional level is a social construct, culture, politics, and societal norms greatly impact professional roles and behavioral concepts. Another challenge exists when examining the microenvironment, such as the clinician-patient interaction. Are norms established by accrediting bodies and patient outcomes sufficient to assess the level of professionalism on the individual and interpersonal constructs of the members of a professional group?

Looking at professionalism from the micro level (individual) through the macro level (societal/institution) gives us varied perspectives to examine situations throughout our professional life. When situations arise that require us to reflect on our own actions and the actions of others, it is helpful to step back and examine the situation from different perspectives. Likewise, as we move into the case studies within this book and as you engage in your professional journey, remember the eight principles of professionalism presented by the Ottawa 2010 conference as a framework.

● MEASURING PROFESSIONALISM

Measuring at the Individual Level (Self-Assessment and Tools Focused on Traits and Attributes)

Measuring professionalism from an individual lens is potentially the most concrete and easiest to envision. Because the individual lens focuses on specific traits and attributes of the person, whether innate or developed, these traits and attributes are measurable through specific evaluation tools. In fact, research shows that there are more than eighty different assessment tools focused on measuring professionalism in health care.[6] The assessment tools vary based on the profession, culture, and setting. Therefore, choosing a reliable and valid assessment that reflects individual characteristics that impact your specific role is important. For example, when comparing allied health professions (physical therapy, occupational therapy, and speech-language pathology), and student professional behaviors, each profession utilizes a different assessment tool. Although these tools share some common themes, they each vary slightly. The differences in assessment tools arise from the history of the profession as well as differing expectations placed on the individual profession in today's health care environment.

A challenge created by relying solely on individual assessment of the attributes of professionalism is this narrowed focus falls short in finding a way to bring together all of the attributes of professionalism into one concise measure of the concept. For example, professional behavior assessments may point to specific strengths and weaknesses but do not bring these strengths and weaknesses together in a summative manner that may influence interactions at the interpersonal level.

Although challenges exist with tools used to measure professionalism through the individual lens, they provide value by providing a means of self-reflection and establishing foundational goals for personal development.

Measuring at the Interpersonal Level (Feedback, Environmental Factors)

Measuring professionalism from the interpersonal level is by far the most daunting. To measure professionalism from this lens, the evaluator should consider the cognitive problem-solving abilities as well as have an understanding of the contextual aspects of the situation, including the setting of the interactions, the role of others involved in an interaction, and the expected outcomes of the situation. Although a more challenging assessment of professionalism, this lens provides a comprehensive summative assessment of professionalism in a specific context. This type of evaluation allows for ongoing dialogue and reflection.

Gaining the broader skills associated with assessing professionalism from an interpersonal lens is important in professional development. Those who learn to incorporate the contextual aspects of the situation with an understanding of the individual's problem-solving abilities become proficient at identifying situations in which professional lapses occur, and can develop corrective strategies.

Measuring at the Societal Level (Accrediting Guidelines, Patient Outcomes, Satisfaction Tools)

Measuring professionalism at a societal or institutional level brings together some of the concrete expectations of individual measures with contextual levels of the interpersonal level. Societal-level measures define specific actions and outcomes of the collective profession or groups of professions in a specific context. For example, accrediting bodies for health care organizations and programs, such as the Joint Commission, provide employee professional engagement criteria. Through this process, we examine the collective action of professionals. Although some individuals may vary in the strengths of professional attributes and examples of a lapse in professionalism may exist within the organization, as a whole, the group may still meet the criteria of professionalism established by the accrediting body.

Another example of measuring professionalism at the societal level is the measure of specific patient outcomes directly impacted by the professionalism of the health care providers engaging with patients. Here again, a specific incident of a lapse in professionalism may not significantly impact a measure of professionalism of the collective.

This level of measure plays an important role in our ability to understand professionalism in health care. By having societal/institutional level measures of professionalism, we establish a collective understanding of the roles and responsibilities of professions. These guiding principles help to define important organizational documents such as a code of conduct or departmental policies and procedures for patient interactions. These societal/institutional-level measures also communicate certain expectations to the patient/consumer. Knowing an organization meets the specific criteria of an accrediting body or obtains specific outcome measures communicates to others the level of professional expectations for the institution's members. In these ways, societal/institutional measures of professionalism play an important role in establishing clear expectations of the collective members.

THE FUTURE OF PROFESSIONALISM

At the beginning of this chapter, we introduced the conundrum of defining professionalism, particularly professionalism for those known as the healers in society. Historically, humans grappled with the concept of professionalism. However, throughout history, we recognized the need to define certain standards or guiding principles by which to inform the expectations of health professionals. As we move through the 21st century, we face our own challenges that shape how we define and assess the health care professions. On a societal level, cultures, technological advancements, political environments, and world events such as the COVID-19 pandemic influence patient outcomes, accreditation standards, and other professional concepts. From an interpersonal perspective, the physical environments in which we engage our patients and colleagues are rapidly changing. For example, remote patient services add an environmental complexity not experienced by health care providers in other centuries. At an individual level, societal diversity and generational norms guide perspectives on individual characteristics and traits and their roles in professionalism.

These factors combine to create the ever-evolving and changing definition and guiding principles of professionalism. Therein lies the conundrum of professionalism. Professionalism is not a static concept that one learns early in their education and applies throughout their career. The study and growth of professionalism must be a lifelong endeavor in which one must willingly reflect and reevaluate ideas and principles to integrate new concepts and ideas as the world evolves. This book is structured to give you basic concepts and applications to professionalism in the 21st century. It is also structured to give you a framework of personal strategic development to utilize as a tool for lifelong professional development.

SUMMARY

In this chapter, we explored the conundrum of defining professionalism in health care. Examining professionalism through its historical context, we see how it is an evolving concept whose meaning continues to change as we gain new perspectives on the ways in which humans interact. Through time, things such as technological advancements, cultural changes, and our deeper understanding of how our bodies and minds process the world have shaped our understanding of what professionalism means. Since professionalism may be approached differently by different professions, we will focus on professionalism in physical therapy for the remainder of this text. As you read through the following chapters of this book, remember professionalism's long history and the complexity of understanding the concept through the individual, interpersonal, and societal lens. Having this foundation gives the reader an understanding that each of the concepts discussed in this book is fluid and evolving, not only for you individually but for all of us as a collective society. Returning to this book for a review of the concepts throughout your career will help to ground your thinking of how you and the profession evolve in understanding professionalism.

Reflection Moment

The next chapters will examine the history and guiding documents of professionalism within physical therapy. Part 2 of this book will then introduce what we feel are common tenets and provide case studies that allow the reader to gain insight into how context defines professionalism. Each chapter of this book ends with an opportunity to self-reflect and gain insight into your professional development as an emerging, reflective, or influencing professional. Reflecting at the end of each chapter and writing the answers to the questions provided allows the ability to formulate an understanding of your current level of development and create a plan for future growth. This book will help you create a concrete plan for professional growth. This is helpful as a student, an early career professional, and as a returning practicing clinician. Going through these exercises throughout your career creates a lifelong learning process for professional development. Please take a few moments to reflect on the two questions below and write down your thoughts:

1. Consider your current perspective of professionalism. Do you focus primarily on one aspect (individual, interpersonal, societal)?
   A. If so, why?
   B. How can you expand your perspectives to use all three lenses?
2. Have you examined your own level of professionalism in the past?
   A. If no, how might you start?
   B. If yes, what tools or strategies have you used to measure your professionalism?

References

1. Applebee G. A brief history of medical professionalism—and why professionalism matters. *Contemp Pediatr.* 2006;23(10):53-62.
2. Bhavana KR, Shreevathsa. Medical geography in Charaka Samhita. *Ayu.* 2014;35(4):371-377. doi:10.4103/0974-8520.158984.
3. Project Professionalism. Published online 1998. https://medicinainternaucv.files.wordpress.com/2013/02/project-professionalism.pdf. Accessed January 29, 2022.
4. Anderson DK, Irwin KE. Self-assessment of professionalism in physical therapy education. *Work.* 2013;44(3):275-281. doi:10.3233/WOR-121504.
5. Jotkowitz AB, Glick S, Porath A. A physician charter on medical professionalism: A challenge for medical education. *Eur J Intern Med.* 2004;15(1):5-9. doi:10.1016/j.ejim.2003.11.002.
6. Hodges BD, Ginsburg S, Cruess R, et al. Assessment of professionalism: Recommendations from the Ottawa 2010 Conference. *Med Teach.* 2011;33(5):354-363. doi:10.3109/0142159X.2011.577300.

chapter 2

Professionalism in Physical Therapy

To understand a profession, it is vital to consider its history: Wars, epidemics, and legislative advancements have all shaped the physical therapy profession and impacted current practice. This section briefly discusses key historical events that shaped physical therapy practice and the evolution of physical therapy from a technical role to a doctoring profession.

● HISTORY OF PHYSICAL THERAPY – THE BIRTH OF A PROFESSION

As a medicinal application, physical therapy traces its roots back to ancient Greece and the father of medicine, Hippocrates. Ancient Greeks understood the importance of exercise to heal the body and hydrotherapy as a healing modality.[1] Although these practices existed in some form for centuries, it was not until the late 1700s that the modern concepts of physical therapy started to form. The origins of the practice of physiotherapy began in Germany, Sweden, and the Netherlands. These earlier practitioners understood the role of gymnastics, manual therapy, massage, and hydrotherapy in healing and strengthening the body. A few key individuals shaped these early practices.[2-4]

The first formal aspect of physical therapy came in the way of medical gymnastics. Pehr Henrik Ling (1776-1839) is considered the pioneer of physical education and the father of Swedish massage. He created Ling's Central Gymnastics Institute to train medical gymnasts and treat patients with exercise, massage, and manipulation. A few years later, in Germany (1851), the term *physiotherapie* first appeared in a medical journal. Over the next few decades, physiotherapy continued to take shape in Europe, as referenced in several medical journals and practices throughout the Netherlands, Germany, and England.[2,3]

In the United States, the role of physical therapy and the application of exercise, massage, and manipulation found its origins in two paths. First, during the polio epidemic of the early 20th century, restorative aides, primarily women, realized the importance of manual muscle testing and muscle reeducation for individuals diagnosed with polio and made great progress in providing rehabilitation to restore quality of life. The second path grew from the US Army's recognition of the need to rehabilitate soldiers with disabilities. In 1917, the Army developed the Division of Physical Reconstruction and trained people from the physical education professions to work as reconstruction aides. After the outbreak of WWI, the Army developed two areas of focus for reconstruction aides. The first group worked with physicians to provide exercise, hydrotherapy, and massage. This group became the foundation for physical therapy in the United States. The second group worked within the almshouses and insane asylums to provide vocational training. This group was the foundation for occupational therapy in the United States.[2,4-6]

Two women, in particular, were instrumental in the success of the reconstruction aide programs and later in the foundation of the physical therapy profession. Marguerite Sanderson worked as the division director of reconstruction aides at Walter Reed Medical Center, where she trained and deployed reconstruction aides for WWI. Mary McMillan, an English woman who received education in corrective exercise, neuro-anatomy, neurology, and psychology, joined Marguerite as a reconstructive aide in 1918. Together, they began Walter Reed's first physiotherapy department, moving the physical therapy profession in the United States to new levels of expertise and recognition.[4-6]

By 1919, programs employing reconstruction and restorative aides expanded across the United States, with more than 45 hospitals employing more than 700 individuals, primarily women. As the profession grew, so did the need for professional organizations, and by 1920, many local grassroots associations existed. These grassroots associations decided to form the American Women's Physiotherapy Association (AWPTA). On January 15, 1921, the AWPTA held its first official meeting to establish its constitution, professional and scientific standards, elect officers, and establish guidelines for membership. Mary McMillan was elected president through a mail-in vote. This year was a productive one for both the association and Mary. The AWPTA released its first publication, *The PT Review*, on March 1, 1921, and Mary McMillan published her first textbook, *Massage and Therapeutic Exercise for Physiotherapists*. In 1922, the association voted to change its name to be more inclusive of male reconstruction aides and established the American Physiotherapy Association (APA). Later, the association would change its name to the American Physical Therapy Association (APTA).[4–6]

From the early 1920s to the end of the century, the physical therapy profession began to take shape with ever-expanding roles and areas of practice. The scope of this textbook is not to provide a comprehensive summary of the historical context which shaped the profession. However, some key items are worth noting. Wars throughout the century, including World War II, the Korean War, and the Vietnam War, expanded the scope and practice of physical therapy. Legislative changes such as the 1946 Hill-Burton Act, which expanded the role of physical therapists in the hospital, the enactment of Medicare and Medicaid in 1965, and the Social Security Act of 1967, which defined outpatient physical therapy services, are all examples of ways in which legislation shaped the profession of physical therapy. Throughout the 1900s, the APTA, state associations, and state boards continued to move the profession forward by creating state practice acts, licensing examinations, accreditation of academic programs, and more stringent degree requirements. For example, in 1954, the APTA developed the first seven-hour competency examination available to state licensing boards. By 1959, 45 states and the territory of Hawaii had practice acts.

The educational requirements for physical therapists have evolved from two years of training to a bachelor's degree in the 1960s and then in the 1990s to a master's degree, followed by a transition to the clinical doctorate known as the DPT in 2005.

The role and impact of the Physical Therapist Assistant (PTA) cannot be overlooked. By the 1960s it was becoming clear that there were too few PTs to meet the growing demand. While PT aides existed, exploration began to find ways to create support professionals with therapy-specific training. In 1964, the APTA developed the *Ad Hoc Committee to Study the Utilization and Training of Nonprofessional Assistants*. This committee examined the training, tasks, responsibilities, and education of this new practitioner level and established guidelines for the PT/PTA relationship. In 1969, fifteen students graduated from Miami Dade College in Florida and St. Mary's Campus of the College of St. Catherine in Minnesota as the first PTAs. Currently, the educational training for PTAs is two years (five semesters) and includes both didactic and clinical education, similar to PT education. PTAs can also benefit from advanced proficiency pathways and specialty content coursework.

Each progression through history has demonstrated a higher level of responsibility, autonomy, and professionalism in the expanded field of physical therapy. Within the PT/PTA relationship, the PT maintains control of the patient/client management model and is legally and ethically responsible for the supervision and direction of the PTA. However, the PTA is an integral asset to the care of patients and clients. The PT/PTA relationship is one that both grapples with and benefits from a clear understanding of professionalism. Throughout the rest of this chapter, we explore how the physical therapy profession defines and measures professionalism.[4,7]

Defining Professionalism in Physical Therapy

Like other medical professions in the late 1900s, physical therapy practitioners were struggling with what it meant to be a professional in physical therapy. The profession was evolving its educational requirements and expanding clinically. What did all this mean about physical therapists' commitment to their patients, health care practice, and society? How did these expanding roles influence the expectations of practitioners and students? These questions led educators, professionals, and the professional association on a journey to further define and measure professionalism in physical therapy.

Chapter 1 points to the complex and evolving nature of professionalism in health care, so it's no surprise that the field of physical therapy also follows an ever-evolving path of exploring, defining, and measuring professionalism. It is important to consider how the framework and definitions of professionalism developed and how they currently influence the profession.

When defining professionalism, physical therapy looked to the medical model as a framework. A 2002 article in the *Journal of American Medical Association* defined professionalism as "the habitual and judicious use of communication, knowledge, technical skills, clinical reasoning, emotions, values, and reflection in daily practice for the benefit of the individual and community being served."[8,9] In examination of this definition as it applied to physical therapy and particularly how it applied to generational changes in the expectations of professionals in physical therapy, a 2007 article in the *Journal of Physical Therapy Education* further expanded upon this definition. The expanded definition included "communication, loyalty, membership, participation in professional organizations, appropriate dress, mannerisms, respect, behavior toward peers, patients, and those in authority, and work habits such as time management and stress management."[8,9] This definition gives insight into the complex nature of understanding what it means to act professionally in different situations and settings. So, if the definition is complex and the concepts are ever-evolving, how do we determine professionalism? This is where core documents that further examine and define these areas, tools that help dissect the components, and personal reflections all come together to provide physical therapists with the necessary skills to discern professionalism in their practice.

The late 20th century and the early 21st century were busy times in the evolution of professionalism in physical therapy. Educators and clinicians alike recognized the need to more formally define and measure the expectations of the physical therapy profession from an individual, interpersonal, and societal level. From this grew several guiding documents that molded the current understanding of expected qualities in the field of physical therapy. The next sections guide you through these documents and how they evolved to the current measurement standards for professionalism in physical therapy.

Code of Ethics

Throughout the 1900s, as the profession of physical therapy worked to understand its role in the health care system, including the profession's autonomy as well as its interaction with other disciplines, several key documents were developed. In 1935, the APA published the first Code of Ethics and Discipline for the profession. This important document gives insight into the profession's foundation and the long journey that would lie ahead for the evolution of physical therapy to a doctoring profession. The 1935 Code of Ethics outlined the requirements for a physician's diagnosis and referral for physical therapy but also denounced advertising of physical therapy services or dissension from a physician's oversight for procedure or treatment. The Code of Ethics for the APTA would undergo several revisions throughout the 1900s as the profession expanded practice and pushed toward autonomy. For example, from 1973 until 1991, the APTA revised the Code of Ethics five times, demonstrating the evolving dynamic nature of the physical therapy profession. The most current APTA Code of Ethics for the Physical Therapist and the Standards of Ethical Conduct of the Physical Therapist Assistant adopted in 2010 demonstrate the advanced practice expectations of the physical therapy profession. See **Table 2.1** below.[10]

TABLE 2.1. Comparison of 1935 Code of Ethics with the 2010 Code of Ethics for Physical Therapists and 2010 Standards of Ethical Conduct for the Physical Therapist Assistant[10,11]

1935 Code of Ethics for the Physical Therapist	2010 Code of Ethics for Physical Therapists	2010 Standards of Ethical Conduct for the Physical Therapist Assistant
Professional Practice (a) Diagnosing, stating the prognosis of a case, and prescribing of treatment shall be entirely the responsibility of the physician. Any assumptions of this responsibility by one of our members shall be considered unethical. (b) The patient shall be referred back to the physician for periodical examinations. (c) A member shall not attempt to criticize the physician or dictate techniques or procedures.	**Principle No. 1:** Physical Therapists shall respect the inherent dignity and rights of all individuals. 1A. Physical therapists shall act in a respectful manner toward each person regardless of age, gender, race, nationality, religion, ethnicity, social or economic status, sexual orientation, health condition, or disability. 1B. Physical therapists shall recognize their personal biases and shall not discriminate against others in physical therapist practice, consultation, education, research, and administration.	**Standard No. 1:** Physical therapist assistants shall respect the inherent dignity, and rights, of all individuals. 1A. Physical therapist assistants shall act in a respectful manner toward each person regardless of age, gender, race, nationality, religion, ethnicity, social or economic status, sexual orientation, health condition, or disability. 1B. Physical therapist assistants shall recognize their personal biases and shall not discriminate against others in the provision of physical therapist services.
Advertising (a) Members shall not procure patients by means of solicitors, agents, circulars, displays, or advertisements inserted in commercial periodicals. (b) Business cards and announcements in medical journals not stating fees are permissible. A statement that the work is medically supervised should appear on the announcement.	**Principle No. 2:** Physical therapists shall be trustworthy and compassionate in addressing the rights and needs of patients and clients. 2A. Physical therapists shall adhere to the core values of the profession and shall act in the best interests of patients and clients over the interests of the physical therapist. 2B. Physical therapists shall provide physical therapy services with compassionate and caring behaviors that incorporate the individual and cultural differences of patients and clients. 2C. Physical therapists shall provide the information necessary to allow patients or their surrogates to make informed decisions about physical therapist care or participation in clinical research. 2D. Physical therapists shall collaborate with patients and clients to empower them in decisions about their health care. 2E. Physical therapists shall protect confidential patient and client information and may disclose confidential information to appropriate authorities only when allowed or as required by law.	**Standard No. 2:** Physical therapist assistants shall be trustworthy and compassionate in addressing the rights and needs of patients and clients. 2A. Physical therapist assistants shall act in the best interests of patients and clients over the interests of the physical therapist assistant. 2B. Physical therapist assistants shall provide physical therapist interventions with compassionate and caring behaviors that incorporate the individual and cultural differences of patients and clients. 2C. Physical therapist assistants shall provide patients and clients with information regarding the interventions they provide. 2D. Physical therapist assistants shall protect confidential patient and client information and, in collaboration with the physical therapist, may disclose confidential information to appropriate authorities only when allowed or as required by law.

(Continued)

TABLE 2.1. Comparison of 1935 Code of Ethics with the 2010 Code of Ethics for Physical Therapists and 2010 Standards of Ethical Conduct for the Physical Therapist Assistant[10,11] (*Continued*)

1935 Code of Ethics for the Physical Therapist	2010 Code of Ethics for Physical Therapists	2010 Standards of Ethical Conduct for the Physical Therapist Assistant
Behaviors (a) Members shall not indulge, before patients, in criticism of how doctors, co-workers, or predecessors had handled the case. (b) It is well to bear in mind that our reputation as individuals as a group depends upon professional accomplishments and upon adherence to the standards of our organization.	**Principle No. 3:** Physical therapists shall be accountable for making sound professional judgments. 3A. Physical therapists shall demonstrate independent and objective professional judgment in the patient's or client's best interest in all practice settings. 3B. Physical therapists shall demonstrate professional judgment informed by professional standards, evidence (including current literature and established best practice), practitioner experience, and patient and client values. 3C. Physical therapists shall make judgments within their scope of practice and level of expertise and shall communicate with, collaborate with, or refer to peers or other health care professionals when necessary. 3D. Physical therapists shall not engage in conflicts of interest that interfere with professional judgment. 3E. Physical therapists shall provide appropriate direction of and communication with physical therapist assistants and support personnel.	**Standard No. 3:** Physical therapist assistants shall make sound decisions in collaboration with the physical therapist and within the boundaries established by laws and regulations. 3A. Physical therapist assistants shall make objective decisions in the patient's or client's best interest in all practice settings. 3B. Physical therapist assistants shall be guided by information about best practice regarding physical therapist interventions. 3C. Physical therapist assistants shall make decisions based upon their level of competence and consistent with patient and client values. 3D. Physical therapist assistants shall not engage in conflicts of interest that interfere with making sound decisions. 3E. Physical therapist assistants shall provide physical therapist services under the direction and supervision of a physical therapist and shall communicate with the physical therapist when patient or client status requires modifications to the established plan of care.
Discipline (a) There shall be a national committee or chapter committee on ethics. (b) The national committee shall be composed of a chairman who is a member of the executive committee and two other members appointed by her. (c) The duties of this committee shall be (1) to properly weigh the charge and evidence against the offender, and (2) the warranting of further action to present it to the Executive Committee for final consideration.	**Principle No. 4:** Physical therapists shall demonstrate integrity in their relationships with patients and clients, families, colleagues, students, research participants, other health care providers, employers, payers, and the public. 4A. Physical therapists shall provide truthful, accurate, and relevant information and shall not make misleading representations. 4B. Physical therapists shall not exploit persons over whom they have supervisory, evaluative, or other authority (e.g., patients/clients, students, supervisees, research participants, or employees). 4C. Physical therapists shall not engage in any sexual relationship with any of their patients and clients, supervisees, or students. 4D. Physical therapists shall not harass anyone verbally, physically, emotionally, or sexually. 4E. Physical therapists shall discourage misconduct by physical therapists, physical therapist assistants, and other health care professionals and, when appropriate, report illegal or unethical acts, including verbal, physical, emotional, or sexual harassment, to an appropriate authority with jurisdiction over the conduct. 4F. Physical therapists shall report suspected cases of abuse involving children or vulnerable adults to the appropriate authority, subject to the law.	**Standard No. 4:** Physical therapist assistants shall demonstrate integrity in their relationships with patients and clients, families, colleagues, students, research participants, other health care providers, employers, payers, and the public. 4A. Physical therapist assistants shall provide truthful, accurate, and relevant information and shall not make misleading representations. 4B. Physical therapist assistants shall not exploit persons over whom they have supervisory, evaluative or other authority (e.g., patients and clients, students, supervisees, research participants, or employees). 4C. Physical therapist assistants shall not engage in any sexual relationship with any of their patients and clients, supervisees, or students. 4D. Physical therapist assistants shall not harass anyone verbally, physically, emotionally, or sexually. 4E. Physical therapist assistants shall discourage misconduct by physical therapists, physical therapist assistants, and other health care professionals and, when appropriate, report illegal or unethical acts, including verbal, physical, emotional, or sexual harassment, to an appropriate authority with jurisdiction over the conduct. 4F. Physical therapist assistants shall report suspected cases of abuse involving children or vulnerable adults to the appropriate authority, subject to law.

(*Continued*)

TABLE 2.1. Comparison of 1935 Code of Ethics with the 2010 Code of Ethics for Physical Therapists and 2010 Standards of Ethical Conduct for the Physical Therapist Assistant[10,11] (*Continued*)		
1935 Code of Ethics for the Physical Therapist	**2010 Code of Ethics for Physical Therapists**	**2010 Standards of Ethical Conduct for the Physical Therapist Assistant**
	Principle No. 5: Physical therapists shall fulfill their legal and professional obligations. 5A. Physical therapists shall comply with applicable local, state, and federal laws and regulations. 5B. Physical therapists shall have primary responsibility for the supervision of physical therapist assistants and support personnel. 5C. Physical therapists involved in research shall abide by accepted standards governing the protection of research participants. 5D. Physical therapists shall encourage colleagues with physical, psychological, or substance-related impairments that may adversely impact their professional responsibilities to seek the assistance of counsel. 5E. Physical therapists who have knowledge that a colleague is unable to perform their professional duties with reasonable skill and safety shall report this information to the appropriate authority. 5F. Physical therapists shall provide notice and information about alternatives for obtaining care in the event the physical therapist terminates the provider relationship. At the same time, the patient or client continues to need physical therapist services.	**Standard No. 5:** Physical therapist assistants shall fulfill their legal and ethical obligations. 5A. Physical therapist assistants shall comply with applicable local, state, and federal laws and regulations. 5B. Physical therapist assistants shall support the supervisory role of the physical therapist to ensure quality care and promote patient and client safety. 5C. Physical therapist assistants involved in research shall abide by accepted standards governing protection of research participants. 5D. Physical therapist assistants shall encourage colleagues with physical, psychological, or substance-related impairments that may adversely impact their professional responsibilities to seek assistance or counsel. 5E. Physical therapist assistants who have knowledge that a colleague is unable to perform their professional responsibilities with reasonable skill and safety shall report this information to the appropriate authority.
	Principle No. 6: Physical therapists shall enhance their expertise through the lifelong acquisition and refinement of knowledge, skills, abilities, and professional behaviors. 6A. Physical therapists shall achieve and maintain professional competence. 6B. Physical therapists shall take responsibility for their professional development based on critical self-assessment and reflection on changes in physical therapist practice, education, health care delivery, and technology. 6C. Physical therapists shall evaluate the strength of evidence and applicability of content presented during professional development activities before integrating the content or techniques into practice. 6D. Physical therapists shall cultivate practice environments that support professional development, lifelong learning, and excellence.	**Standard No. 6:** Physical therapist assistants shall enhance their competence through the lifelong acquisition and refinement of knowledge, skills, and abilities. 6A. Physical therapist assistants shall achieve and maintain clinical competence. 6B. Physical therapist assistants shall engage in lifelong learning consistent with changes in their roles and responsibilities and advances in the practice of physical therapy. 6C. Physical therapist assistants shall support practice environments that support career development and lifelong learning.

(Continued)

TABLE 2.1. Comparison of 1935 Code of Ethics with the 2010 Code of Ethics for Physical Therapists and 2010 Standards of Ethical Conduct for the Physical Therapist Assistant[10,11]   (*Continued*)

1935 Code of Ethics for the Physical Therapist	2010 Code of Ethics for Physical Therapists	2010 Standards of Ethical Conduct for the Physical Therapist Assistant
	Principle No. 7: Physical therapists shall promote organizational behaviors and business practices that benefit patients and clients, and society. 7A. Physical therapists shall promote practice environments that support autonomous and accountable professional judgments. 7B. Physical therapists shall seek remuneration as is deserved and reasonable for physical therapist services. 7C. Physical therapists shall not accept gifts or other considerations that influence or give an appearance of influencing their professional judgment. 7D. Physical therapists shall fully disclose any financial interest they have in products or services that they recommend to patients and clients. 7E. Physical therapists shall be aware of charges and shall ensure that documentation and coding for physical therapist services accurately reflect the nature and extent of the services provided. 7F. Physical therapists shall refrain from employment arrangements, or other arrangements, that prevent physical therapists from fulfilling professional obligations to patients and clients.	**Standard No. 7:** Physical therapist assistants shall support organizational behaviors and business practices that benefit patients and clients and society. 7A. Physical therapist assistants shall promote work environments that support ethical and accountable decision-making. 7B. Physical therapist assistants shall not accept gifts or other considerations that influence or give an appearance of influencing their decisions. 7C. Physical therapist assistants shall fully disclose any financial interest they have in products or services that they recommend to patients and clients. 7D. Physical therapist assistants shall ensure that documentation for their interventions accurately reflects the nature and extent of the services provided. 7E. Physical therapist assistants shall refrain from employment arrangements, or other arrangements, that prevent physical therapist assistants from fulfilling ethical obligations to patients and clients.
	Principle No. 8: Physical therapists shall participate in efforts to meet the health needs of people locally, nationally, or globally. 8A. Physical therapists shall provide pro bono physical therapy services or support organizations that meet the health needs of people who are economically disadvantaged, uninsured, and underinsured. 8B. Physical therapists shall advocate to reduce health disparities and health care inequities, improve access to health care services, and address the health, wellness, and preventive health care needs of people. 8C. Physical therapists shall be responsible stewards of health care resources and shall avoid overutilization or under-utilization of physical therapist services. 8D. Physical therapists shall educate members of the public about the benefits of physical therapy and the unique role of the physical therapist.	**Standard No. 8:** Physical therapist assistants shall participate in efforts to meet the health needs of people locally, nationally, or globally. 8A. Physical therapist assistants shall support organizations that meet the health needs of people who are economically disadvantaged, uninsured, and underinsured. 8B. Physical therapist assistants shall advocate for people with impairments, activity limitations, participation restrictions, and disabilities in order to promote their participation in community and society. 8C. Physical therapist assistants shall be responsible stewards of health care resources by collaborating with physical therapists in order to avoid overutilization or underutilization of physical therapist services. 8D. Physical therapist assistants shall educate members of the public about the benefits of physical therapy.

Reflection Moment

Take some time to review Table 2.1 to understand how, in less than 100 years, the profession matured in professionalism and practice and moved toward an awareness of societal accountability and moral responsibility.

- Consider how different our profession would be if we practiced under the 1935 Code of Ethics for Physical Therapists.

- How do the ethical standards inform the professional relationship between the PT and PTA?

From Generic Abilities to Professional Behaviors

In the early 1990s, educators at the University of Wisconsin-Madison set out to establish an assessment of essential behaviors critical to graduate physical therapists' clinical success.

This assessment arose from recognizing that some students struggled to transition from the classroom to the clinic not because of clinical knowledge or skills but from underdeveloped professional behaviors. Although faculty often modeled these behaviors, the coursework did not specifically include them. Faculty at the University of Wisconsin-Madison and volunteer clinicians utilized the Ability-Based Assessment from the medical program at Alverno College in Milwaukee to establish the *Generic Abilities Assessment for Physical Therapy* in 1993. This assessment would become the foundational document for assessing classroom and clinical education professional behaviors through the 1990s and early 2000s.[12]

Through their research, the faculty developed ten generic abilities valued by clinicians who supported students in the clinical education process. The assessment tool divided the generic abilities into three developing levels: beginning, developing, and advanced, and provided written objective descriptions for each level of development within the ten generic abilities. The assessment tool that examined these ten abilities was one of the first formal professionalism assessments in physical therapy and helped move the profession forward in examining the outcomes of physical therapy education. In 2010, the authors updated these definitions and renamed the *Professional Behaviors for the 21st Century* document. Refer to **Table 2.2** to learn more about these ten behaviors.[12,13]

APTA Vision Statement

In 2000, the APTA vision statement for the next twenty years directed strategic change for physical therapy. In this Vision 2020 statement, the APTA outlined six critical elements of the path forward for the profession of physical therapy. These six key elements were direct access, evidence-based practice, professionalism, doctoring profession, autonomous practice, and practitioner of choice.[14] It is essential to note the significant change in the profession from those early ethical guidelines in which the profession relied upon the referral and oversight of a physician to an autonomous, doctoring practitioner striving for patients' ability to have unrestricted direct access to their services. The APTA 2020 Vision set the foundation for the strategic process of moving physical therapy into a doctoring profession.

The physical therapy profession made many strides in achieving the vision set in 2000. By 2005, schools were graduating practitioners, and the profession was well on its way to gaining direct access, thus furthering the autonomous practice of physical therapists nationwide.[15] Therefore, revising the APTA vision once again made sense to reflect the growing autonomy and impact of the profession on society. In 2013, APTA updated the vision statement: "Transforming society by optimizing movement to improve the human experience."* Here again, the widening scope of the profession, autonomy, and expectations

TABLE 2.2. Professional Behaviors for the 21st Century

Professional Behaviors for the 21st Century	Definition
Commitment to Learning	The ability to self-assess, self-correct, and self-direct: to identify needs and sources of learning and continue to seek new knowledge and understanding.
Interpersonal Skills	The ability to interact effectively with patients, families, colleagues, other health care professionals, and the community in a culturally aware manner.
Communication Skills	The ability to communicate effectively (i.e., speaking body language, reading, writing, listening) for varied audiences and purposes.
Effective Use of Time and Resources	The ability to manage time and resources effectively to obtain the maximum possible benefit.
Use of Constructive Feedback	The ability to seek out and identify quality sources of feedback, reflect on and integrate the feedback, and provide meaningful feedback to others.
Problem-solving	The ability to recognize and define problems, analyze data, develop and implement solutions, and evaluate outcomes.
Professionalism	The ability to exhibit appropriate professional conduct and to represent the profession effectively while promoting the growth/development of the Physical Therapy profession.
Responsibility	The ability to be accountable for the outcomes of personal and professional actions and to follow through on commitments that encompass the profession within the scope of work, community and social responsibilities.
Critical Thinking	The ability to question logically; identify, generate and evaluate elements of logical argument; recognize and differentiate facts, appropriate or faulty inferences, and assumptions; and distinguish relevant from irrelevant information. The ability to appropriately utilize, analyze, and critically evaluate scientific evidence to develop a logical argument, and to identify and determine the impact of bias on the decision-making process.
Stress Management	The ability to identify sources of stress and to develop and implement effective coping behaviors; this applies to interactions for self, patient/clients and their families, members of the health care team, and in work/life scenarios.

Reproduced with permission from May, Warren W PT, MPH; Morgan, Barbara J PhD, PT; Lemke, Janet C MA, PT; Karst, Gregory M PhD, PT; Stone, Howard L PhD. Model for Ability-Based Assessment in Physical Therapy Education. J Phys Ther Educ. 1995;9(1): 3-6[12,13]

of those calling themselves physical therapists and physical therapist assistants are evident.[14]

Core Values

The APTA established core values for the physical therapy profession as part of the strategic process. In 2003, the APTA adopted seven core values as their guiding document for professionalism in physical therapy. The APTA modeled the Core Values after the American Board of Internal Medicine's (ABIM) 2002 document, *Medical Professionalism in the New Millennium: A Physician's Charter,* which offered six guiding principles of professionalism in medicine. These six guiding principles held to three key values: (1) altruism, (2) patient autonomy, and (3) social justice. These key values were woven through the seven APTA core values as a common theme. By using the ABIM model as a guiding document for professionalism, the APTA further cemented its dedication to physical therapy as a doctoring profession. The three key values of altruism, patient autonomy, and social justice are evident in the APTA core values. One can also see the threads of the Ottawa conference's framework and eight guiding principles of professionalism as discussed in Chapter 1.[16–18] These core values are instrumental in guiding the individual, interpersonal, and societal professional engagement of physical therapy.

In 2013, the APTA developed *Professionalism in Physical Therapy: Core Values Self-Assessment* to facilitate understanding of these original seven core values. This self-assessment tool allowed clinicians and students to examine the frequency at which they exhibited key components of each core value.[16,19]

As mentioned throughout this textbook, as society advances and we gain a deeper understanding of the world in which we live, professional values and ideals also evolve. Just as the ethical principles and vision statement matured, so too have the APTA Core Values. In 2019, the APTA adopted a revised version of this guiding document. In updating the core values, the APTA aligned the physical therapist and physical therapist assistant under the same guidance values. The nine updated core values reflect an ever-changing society and practice of physical therapy. At the time of this textbook publication, a complementary self-assessment tool for the nine core values is unavailable. However, physical therapists, physical therapist assistants, and students can still apply the original assessment tool designed for 2003 Core Values as a foundation and then consider the additional core values of collaboration and inclusion in their discussions of core values. **Table 2.3** lists the updated nine core values.[20]

Through examination of these guiding documents and reflection on their impact on physical therapy practitioners, the evolution from technician to professional unfolds. The ethical principles, *Professional Behaviors for the 21st Century*, APTA Vision Statement, and the Core Values for the Physical Therapist and Physical Therapist Assistant provide a framework for

TABLE 2.3.   Core Values of the Physical Therapist and Physical Therapist Assistant

Core Value	Definition
Accountability	Accountability is active acceptance of the responsibility for the diverse roles, obligations, and actions of the physical therapist and physical therapist assistant including self-regulation and other behaviors that positively influence patient and client outcomes, the profession, and the health needs of society.
Altruism	Altruism is the primary regard for or devotion to the interest of patients and clients, thus assuming the responsibility of placing the needs of patients and clients ahead of the physical therapist's or physical therapist assistant's self-interest.
Collaboration*	Collaboration is working together with patients and clients, families, communities, and professionals in health and other fields to achieve shared goals. Collaboration within the physical therapist-physical therapist assistant team is working together, within each partner's respective role, to achieve optimal physical therapist services and outcomes for patients and clients.
Compassion and Caring	Compassion is the desire to identify with or sense something of another's experience, a precursor of caring. Caring is the concern, empathy, and consideration for the needs and values of others.
Duty	Duty is the commitment to meeting one's obligations to provide effective physical therapist services to patients and clients, to serve the profession, and to positively influence the health of society.
Excellence	Excellence in the provision of physical therapist services occurs when the physical therapist and physical therapist assistant consistently use current knowledge and skills while understanding personal limits, integrate the patient or client perspective, embrace advancement, and challenge mediocrity.
Inclusion*	Inclusion occurs when the physical therapist and physical therapist assistant create a welcoming and equitable environment for all. Physical therapists and physical therapist assistants are inclusive when they commit to providing a safe space, elevating diverse and minority voices, acknowledging personal biases that may impact patient care, and taking a position of anti-discrimination.
Integrity	Integrity is steadfast adherence to high ethical principles or standards, being truthful, ensuring fairness, following through on commitments, and verbalizing to others the rationale for actions.
Social Responsibility	Social responsibility is the promotion of a mutual trust between the profession and the larger public that necessitates responding to societal needs for health and wellness.

*Denotes core value added to the updated 2019 document.

guiding this profession through the ever-changing health care environment. What patients, communities, and society needed from physical therapists in the last century and even in the last twenty years may differ greatly from future expectations. As you work through the components of the textbook, it's important to keep the historical context as a reference point but also to reflect on the future patient, community, and societal needs that may impact our profession and our practice.

● THE FUTURE OF PROFESSIONALISM IN PHYSICAL THERAPY

In 2014, the American Council of Academic Physical Therapy (ACAPT), in collaboration with the APTA, held a summit focused on exploring the clinical education of physical therapists. This summit catalyzed ongoing engagement on best conducting clinical education as an integral component of preparing new graduate physical therapists and physical therapist assistants as professionals. Some key areas of recommendation of the summit focused on the ongoing development of early, intermittent, and final clinical, and educational core competencies, including professional behaviors. The summit recommendations also included expanding community-centered physical therapist services, which integrate into professional education to meet societal needs. This summit is an example of how the physical therapy profession continues to evolve our role and the level of professionalism needed to strive toward the APTA vision of transforming society through human movement.[14,21]

Although professionalism is considered an important component of individual and group collective identity, the behaviors and skills associated with professionalism are historically considered "soft skills." Recently, the importance of these soft skills to success in the workplace has gained traction. The term "employability skills" often now replaces the term soft skills. By defining these as employability skills, one understands the importance to not only patients and the physical therapy profession but also how it impacts one's livelihood and future within the profession.[22]

● SUMMARY

In this chapter, we examined how the profession of physical therapy advanced from its technician-based origins to the profession of today. Through the historical journey of physical therapy, we gained insight into how critical documents such as the Code of Ethics came into being and evolved to meet the ever-changing needs of patients, the profession, communities, and society. We explored other documents which support not only understanding professionalism in physical therapy but also provide a means by which to measure specific attributes of physical therapy.

Reflection Moment

Consider the guiding principles and documents which frame physical therapy professionalism (Code of Ethics for the Physical Therapist, Standards of Ethical Conduct for the Physical Therapist Assistant, Professional Behaviors for the 21st Century, and the APTA Core Values for the Physical Therapist and Physical Therapist Assistant). Connect these standards, behaviors, and values to the concept of the three levels of professionalism discussed in Chapter 1.

1. How do these documents impact your individual, interpersonal and societal-institutional actions?
2. What do you think of our foundational documents? Do they do a good job of moving our profession and the concept of professionalism forward?
3. Looking ahead toward professional development and growth, are there any standards, behaviors, and values you consider an individual strength? Are there any areas of challenge? Keep these in mind as we move forward.

References

1. Kleisiaris CF, Sfakianakis C, Papathanasiou IV. Health care practices in ancient Greece: The Hippocratic ideal. *J Med Ethics Hist Med*. 2014;7:6-6.
2. Shairk A, Shemzaz A. The rise of physical therapy: A history in footsteps. *Arch Med Health Sci*. 2014;2(2):257-269. doi:10.4103/2321-4848.144367.
3. Terlouw TJA. The origin of the term "physiotherapy." Editorial in Physiotherapy Research International 2005; 10:124-125. *Physiother Res Int*. 2006;11(1):56-57. doi:10.1002/pri.33.
4. Moffat M. The history of physical therapy practice in the United States. *J Phys Ther Educ Am Phys Ther Assoc Educ Sect*. 2003;17(3):15-25.
5. Remembering the Reconstruction Aides. American Physical Therapy Association. Published March 8, 2018. Accessed March 20, 2022. https://www.apta.org/article/2018/03/09/remembering-the-reconstruction-aides.
6. Aguilar A, Stupans I, Scutter S, King S. Exploring professionalism: The professional values of Australian occupational therapists. *Aust Occup Ther J*. 2012;59(3):209-217.
7. Nieland VM, Harris MJ. History of accreditation in physical therapy education. *J Phys Ther Educ*. 2003;17(3). https://journals.lww.com/jopte/Fulltext/2003/10000/History_of_Accreditation_in_Physical_Therapy.7.aspx.
8. Anderson DK, Irwin KE. Self-assessment of professionalism in physical therapy education. *Work*. 2013;44(3):275-281. doi:10.3233/WOR-121504.
9. Gleeson PB. Understanding generational competence related to professionalism: Misunderstandings that lead to a perception of unprofessional behavior. *J Phys Ther Educ*. 2007;21(3). https://journals.lww.com/jopte/Fulltext/2007/10000/Understanding_Generational_Competence_Related_to.4.aspx.
10. Swisher LL, Hiller P, for the APTA Task Force to Revise the Core Ethics Documents. The revised APTA code of ethics for the physical therapist and standards of ethical conduct for the physical therapist assistant: Theory, purpose, process, and significance. *Phys Ther*. 2010;90(5):803-824. doi:10.2522/ptj.20090373.
11. Unknown. 1935 APA adopts a code of ethics and discipline. https://centennial.apta.org/timeline/apa-adopts-a-code-of-ethics-and-discipline/. Accessed March 28, 2022.
12. May WW, Morgan BJ, Lemke JC, Karst GM, Stone HL. Model for ability-based assessment in physical therapy education. *J Phys Ther Educ*. 1995;9(1). https://journals.lww.com/jopte/Fulltext/1995/01000/Model_for_Ability_Based_Assessment_in_Physical.2.aspx.
13. May W, Kontney L, Iglarsh A. Professional behaviors for the 21st century. Published online 2010.

14. Vision statements for the physical therapy profession established. https://centennial.apta.org/timeline/vision-statement-for-the-physical-therapy-profession-established/#:~:text=In%20 2000%2C%20APTA%20was%20focused,path%20forward%20 for%20the%20profession.

15. Levels of patient access to physical therapy services in the US. Published online September 23, 2021. https://www.apta.org/ advocacy/issues/direct-access-advocacy/direct-access-by-state. Accessed April 10, 2022.

16. Anderson D. *A Validation Study of the APTA Professionalism in Physical Therapy Core Values Self-Assessment.* Northern Illinois University; 2015.

17. Hodges BD, Ginsburg S, Cruess R, et al. Assessment of professionalism: Recommendations from the Ottawa 2010 Conference. *Med Teach.* 2011;33(5):354-363. doi:10.3109/0142159X.2011.577300.

18. Project Professionalism. Published online 1998. https://medicinainternaucv.files.wordpress.com/2013/02/project-professionalism.pdf. Accessed January 29, 2022.

19. Professionalism in physical therapy: Cover values self-assessment. https://www.apta.org/contentassets/aec54663ee514f0580449b7ee-59ac18c/core-values-self-assessment.pdf. Accessed April 10, 2022.

20. Core Values for Physical Therapist and Physical Therapist Assistant HOD P09-21-21-09. Published online December 14, 2021. https://www.apta.org/apta-and-you/leadership-and-governance/ policies/core-values-for-the-physical-therapist-and-physical-therapist-assistant. Accessed April 10, 2022.

21. *American Council of Academic Physical Therapy Clinical Education Summit*; 2020.

22. McCallum CA, Murray L, Tilstra M, Lairson A. Assessment of employability skills: A systematic review of the availability and usage of professional behavior assessment instruments. *J Phys Ther Educ.* 2020;34(3). https://journals.lww.com/jopte/Fulltext/2020/09000/ Assessment_of_Employability_Skills__A_Systematic.12.aspx.

chapter 3

Professionalism: A Working Model

To this point, we have explored the meaning of professionalism and how physical therapy has integrated the core concepts of professionalism into its practice as it evolved from its technical roots to today's profession. In this chapter, we establish a working model for you to explore your professional development. This framework builds on the principles from the Ottawa Conference and the core documents of physical therapy professionalism; APTA Core Values, Professional Behaviors for the 21st Century, APTA ethical principles, and APTA Vision Statement.

This chapter defines three levels of professional development: emerging, reflective, and influencing, using an oak tree analogy. These levels flow through the remainder of the book as we explore concepts of professionalism. Review these three levels periodically and reflect on which best describes your thoughts in the case scenarios and reflection questions at the end of each chapter in Part 2 of this book.

We use these levels of professionalism and the oak tree analogy to provide a framework for self-reflection to create a working model for your professional development. By using reflection, we help develop a strategic thinking process to guide you in developing professional goals, tactics, and measures of success.

In this chapter, we also briefly outline seven concepts of professionalism that connect self-reflection to growth toward your strategic professional development. Part 2 of this book covers the seven concepts in depth and provides reflective activities to allow further self-exploration. Part 3 of this book then builds on your strategic thinking reflections to guide you in creating your strategic professional development plan.

● THE OAK TREE ANALOGY FOR PROFESSIONAL GROWTH

The oak tree provides a powerful analogy when considering your professional growth. This analogy has long been used to symbolize growth, strength, and steadiness but also symbolizes that these traits have humble beginnings. The tall oak grows

from an acorn to a sapling and then to one of the hardiest trees in the forest. As the oak tree adds rings to its trunk and limbs to its span, it gains strength. It adapts and becomes more resilient to the challenges that surround it. This analogy is synonymous with professional development.

As a new or emerging clinician, you are like the acorn. You have the necessary ingredients to function as a physical therapist, and with the right environment, care, and time, you also can strengthen your professionalism with upward and outward growth. As you evolve in your career and gain experiences, seek out mentorship, and add strategies to your clinical problem-solving, you become more like a sapling, a reflective clinician. As a reflective clinician, you gain trust in yourself and your environment; your growth in critical thinking, problem-solving, and engagement set strong roots for continued strength and stability in your professional development. Navigation of this phase is critical to maturity and development. The rate, level, and time to maturity depend on many factors, but it is in this intermediate phase that roots are established.

With nurturing, eventually, you gain attributes of the grand oak tree. With maturity, the influencing clinician becomes confident in professional practices and mentoring others. This influence and professional maturity have the capacity to impact the character, development, and behavior of others. But at the same time, just as the oak tree continues to add rings and branches, an influencing professional recognizes the responsibility to continue to grow, learn, and strengthen professionalism. This is your lifelong journey. Picture the oak tree and the emerging, reflective, and influencing clinician definitions listed below to frame your thinking as you step into the next chapters of this book.

 EMERGING PROFESSIONAL

This level is where most physical therapy students/practitioners begin their journey. It is the entry-level awareness of the importance of personal behaviors and their impact on professional growth and opportunity. It reflects the understanding of self and the desire to manifest or develop the necessary skills to develop as a respected professional.

REFLECTING PROFESSIONAL

This level denotes a student/practitioner who is reflective of interactions and deliberate in response. It denotes a level of growth and maturity that is responsive to contemplation and feedback. This level is necessary to develop as a professional capable of leading others.

INFLUENCING PROFESSIONAL

This is the pinnacle of professionalism and denotes a practitioner who understands their role and responsibility as a model for others. They mentor others toward growth and development in their profession with an understanding that maturing as a professional is an ongoing, interactive process.

As you read through the following chapters, think about how core values and professional behaviors evolve as you move through these levels. For example, how might an emerging professional communicate to a patient, family member, or peer differently than an influencing professional? What skills and strategies do we gain throughout our professional life that refine these behaviors? How do we seek out learning opportunities and experiences to improve these behaviors? By actively reflecting on these concepts in the early phase of your career, you develop a purpose-driven approach to your professional development. Instead of relying on chance opportunities and encounters, you guide your professional development with meaning and focus.

● STRATEGIC THINKING FOR PROFESSIONAL DEVELOPMENT

Strategic thinking refers to analyzing situations from a broad perspective using a structured framework to understand the potential opportunities for the best future decisions.[1] As a physical therapist or a physical therapist assistant, you apply critical thinking skills to each patient's daily care plan. For example, the collection of objective medical data, assessment of the relationship between medical data and an individual's quality of life, collaboration to set patient goals, and determination of a plan of action all reflect the same skill set necessary to think strategically about professional interactions.

Previously, we discussed three ways to view professionalism: individual, interpersonal, and societal. These perspectives provide a framework for strategic thinking in professional development. When considering your professional development, you can reflect on ways in which you can view your professional growth through these three lenses. First, by examining it through careful reflection that leads to the personal development of specific behaviors and actions (individual); second, by surveying your current environment, creating awareness of individual differences to understand the impact of social engagement in defining professionalism in that setting (interpersonal); third,

by understanding the societal expectations and role of your profession to amplify your potential (societal). In doing this exercise, you help to formulate a strategic plan for your professional growth. You can set goals for your behaviors, goals for engaging in your workplace to create the highest level of professionalism in the environment and, finally, goals for advocacy to further the scope and level of the profession of physical therapy in society. Building on these objectives, you can develop specific daily actions and tactics that can lead to growth in professional development and maturity. Finally, you can establish key measures of success and timeframes to ensure you are moving toward achieving the established goals.

● CONCEPTS IN PROFESSIONALISM

The Ottawa Conference provides eight principles to guide our thinking about professionalism. Likewise, the APTA ethics principles provide eight principles to guide ethical decision-making in the practice of physical therapy, and the APTA core values and the Professional Behaviors for the 21st Century provide guiding areas to focus on professional development. Understanding these documents and their guidance is an essential step in professional development. Physical therapists and physical therapist assistants should have these documents readily available to reference and reflect on as opportunities for professional development arise. For this book, we used these documents to guide our understanding of a few areas of professional development applicable to understanding professionalism through individual, interpersonal, and societal lenses. These areas outlined below are not an all-inclusive list of professionalism but rather a way to organize your thinking around the many facets of professional growth.

The goal of this book is to provide a framework for professionalism and guidance on strategic thinking for professional growth. The areas covered in the next sections of the book connect professional and personal development through self-reflection activities that encourage strategic thinking. While the physical therapy guiding documents provide a foundation for professional growth, reality and experience will deepen these core traits into behaviors that will ultimately shape you professionally. The following seven concepts in professionalism were chosen because they represent areas that influence individual, interpersonal, and societal interactions; and, when incorporated into a strategic growth plan, will impact personal and professional development. Thoughtful reflection on these concepts will provide insight into your current practices and provide avenues to mature as an influencing professional.

Communication

Effective communication is one of the most important skills for success. Health care professionals require a higher level of communication strategies than most other professions. In health care, one needs to have flexibility in communication to effectively translate complex medical terminology and concepts to those outside of health care, effectively communicate with other health care disciplines who may not be familiar with specific discipline concepts, and communicate with a variety of businesses that connect to health care. Therefore, it is important to understand how communication works, from the basic framework of communication to the many different ways humans communicate with each other.

Emotional Intelligence

Emotional Intelligence consists of three specific components: self, others, and motivation. This learned behavior allows us to be aware of and manage our own emotions as well as have awareness of the emotions of others. As we gain skills in this area, we also gain an ability to focus on goals and tasks at hand regardless of our own emotional state and the emotional environment of those around us. Consider how powerful this skill is in professional development within the health care environment. For example, clinicians with strong emotional intelligence can support themselves and others in navigating life-altering events, staying focused during emergency situations, and plotting a course toward positive results during times of high emotional turmoil.[2-4]

Resilience and Grit

Resilience and grit are often interchanged. Resilience is the ability to recover from difficulties or challenges, whereas grit is the toughness to keep pushing through challenges. You probably can see why these two terms are often interchanged. In the health care environment, clinicians face many difficult situations which require the skills to keep working through the situation and to recover from the trauma the situation may cause. There is significant research on how humans gain resilience and grit and why some are more resilient or gritty than others. In the chapter on this topic, we explore the literature regarding this valuable skill and discuss ways to build resilience and grit throughout your career.[5-7]

Accountability

Accountability begins with accepting the current reality of the situation. Once we accept the situation, we can determine the next actionable steps. Although this may seem obvious and even simple, there are many examples in our own lives where we fall into the trap of blaming others, finding excuses, or even denying a situation exists. As health care professionals, there are many incidents in which we must state the current situation and determine decisive action to ensure the health and well-being of others. Here again, as we develop our accountability strategies and move toward the influencing clinician, we gain a strong sense of accountability and an understanding that recognizing the current situation and taking action not only benefits our patients and ourselves but helps to build a strong foundation for all members of the health care team.

Cultural Quotient

Cultural intelligence builds upon emotional intelligence. As we develop our skills in understanding ourselves and supporting others, we need to integrate the understanding of cultural nuances which influences how we engage in interpersonal situations and respond to societal changes. In the chapter on this topic, we explore our motivation for cultural intelligence, ways to expand our cultural knowledge, and strategies to process our culturally diverse experiences into professional growth.[8]

Social Responsibility

A core value of the APTA, social responsibility demonstrates our profession's commitment to societal needs. This attribute guides each professional in understanding their role outside the walls of the health care facility. By exploring your connection to social responsibility, you gain a deeper appreciation for the roles that you play in improving the health and wellness of not just the patients who enter the health care system but of your community and society as a whole. As we move from emerging to influencing clinicians, we learn to connect each and every action we take as health care professionals to contribute to society, and we mentor those around us to understand the interconnectedness of our actions both inside the clinic setting and in our day-to-day lives.

Management of Self through Lifelong Learning

Management of self or self-management is a term that is often used but poorly understood. What does it mean to manage yourself? There are many areas where we can consider self-management, such as in our everyday actions, personal and professional life, interactions with others, or even behaviors when no one is watching. Management of self has a strong relationship with emotional intelligence, ethics, and core values and requires daily reflection. It is also strongly connected to lifelong learning. After completing many years of formal education, physical therapy professionals enter the workforce with the basic recipe to provide competent patient care. However, this is only the beginning of the journey. Graduate physical therapists and physical therapist assistants quickly learn that there are still many behaviors, skills, and techniques that will benefit from continued development. Lifelong learning not only applies to hands-on skills but also to the continued learning and understanding of the role we play in our communities and society. As we get into the routine of everyday working life, it is easy to put off our learning process for other more pressing daily life activities. To continue to develop as professionals, we need to commit to self-management and lifelong learning. This commitment is not only about the integration of new evidence and skills into practice but also about the development of our interpersonal skills and how to engage the practice of physical therapy in the community and society as a whole.

● SUMMARY

In this chapter, we defined the oak tree analogy of professional growth through emerging, reflective, and influencing levels of professionalism. We introduced strategic thinking and the eight concepts of professionalism. The oak tree analogy, strategic thinking strategies, and the eight concepts provide the tools for self-reflective professional development.

Reflection Moment

Consider the Oak Tree Model of Professional Growth and its three stages. Choose two of the concepts in professionalism and take a few minutes to answer the following questions:

1. For the two concepts of professionalism you chose, from your current understanding of these areas, do you

consider yourself as an emerging, reflective, or influencing professional? Why?

2. For the two concepts of professionalism you chose, what is one goal you could set to expand your growth in that area? How might you work to achieve this goal? What would success in that concept look like to you?

References

1. Nina Bowman. *HBR Guide to Thinking Strategically, See the Big Picture, Focus on What Matters, Make Smarter Decisions Chapter 3: Prove you're ready for the next level by showing off your strategic thinking skills.* Harvard Business School Publishing Corporation; 2019.

2. Goleman D. *Emotional Intelligence: Why It Can Matter More than IQ. 10th Anniversary Edition.* Banton Books; 2005.

3. Pienimaa A, Haavisto E, Talman K. Emotional intelligence instruments used in health care education. *J Nurs Educ.* 2022;61(1):6-11. doi:10.3928/01484834-20211130-01.

4. Roth CG, Eldin KW, Padmanabhan V, Friedman EM. Twelve tips for the introduction of emotional intelligence in medical education. *Med Teach.* 2019;41(7):746-749. doi:10.1080/0142159X.2018.1481499.

5. Duckworth A. *Grit: The Power of Passion and Perseverance.* Scribner; 2016.

6. Calo M, Judd B, Chipchase L, Blackstock F, Peiris CL. Grit, resilience, mindset, and academic success in physical therapist students: A cross-sectional, multicenter study. *Phys Ther.* 2022;102(6):pzac038. doi:10.1093/ptj/pzac038.

7. Zolli A, Healy AM. *Resilience: Why Things Bounce Back.* Simon & Schuster Paperbacks; 2012.

8. Livermore D. *Leading with Cultural Intelligence: The New Secret to Success.* American Management Association; 2010.

PART

2

CONCEPTS IN PROFESSIONALISM

Refer to this section to explore the individual components
that are essential to growth as a professional

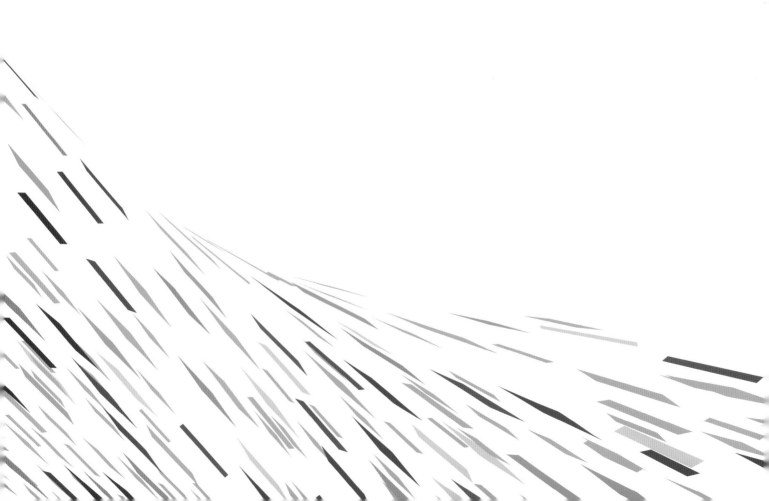

chapter 4

Communication

Professional communication plays a critical role in health care. Health care professionals must communicate effectively with patients, their families, other professionals, and community members. To effectively communicate, health care professionals must adapt communication to their audience and understand the many ways humans interact. In this chapter, we explore communication models, how communication varies based on the audience, the development of communication as professional behavior, and the impact of effective communication in health care.[1]

What is the first thing that comes to mind when you think of communication? You may think of a conversation with a friend or colleague or about communication via email or text. However, communication is a complex web of many components: verbal interactions, written interactions, how we move, the environment, and our personal history and experiences.[2] An effective communicator understands how each of the components potentially influences the conversation. As we explore communication in more detail, it helps to understand some foundational concepts. The first section of this chapter outlines these concepts.

● MODELS OF COMMUNICATION

The development of models regarding how we communicate began in the late 1940s when the expansion of communication technology increased the complexity of human interaction. Understanding the models as a framework for today's complex communications is essential. Let's explore three communication models: linear, interactional, and transactional.

The linear communication model developed in the late 1940s influenced most of the thinking around how communication worked for most of the 20th century. This model is basic in design, consisting of a sender, a receiver, and a message. According to this model, communication has a distinct beginning and end and travels in one direction from the sender to the receiver. Although this model accounts for disruption in the message, referred to as noise, it misses many other complexities of communication, such as listening, and the ongoing interaction between the sender and listener.[2]

Consider how basic our communication looks when we simply send a message, someone passively receives this message, and then we repeat the process. Email and text are perfect examples of the linear model of communication. If you have ever experienced frustration from an email or text, it is likely because it was missing the components that make communication a rich experience. While ignoring the many complexities of communication, the linear model provides a foundation for considering communication, including the understanding that the message contains several components. **Figure 4.1** demonstrates the basic linear communication model.[2]

The Interactional communication model expands upon the linear model by adding a feedback channel, thus providing a two-channel mode. In this mode, a sender provides a message, and the receiver processes the message and provides feedback either verbally or nonverbally. Another essential component of the interactional communication model is the field of experience for both the sender and the receiver. The field of experience explains how we construct and interact with the message based on our culture, environment, cognition, and lived experiences. This model dramatically expands on the linear model, recognizing comprehension and personal experience's role in the interaction. Finally, this model acknowledges that the same person often acts as both a sender and receiver but falls short of explaining that someone can simultaneously be a sender and receiver. So, let's dig a bit deeper into the nuances of this model. In the linear model, a sender sends a message, which may interfere with the transmission, the message connects to the receiver, and the transaction is complete. In the interactional model,

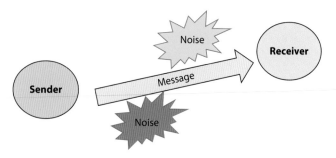

FIGURE 4.1. Linear Model of Communication.

we see that initially, the sender frames the message through their own experiences before sending it. The message travels to the receiver, who also frames it through their lived experiences. The receiver responds by providing feedback framed through both individuals' experiences. We see how communication becomes more complex in that we change the message by our perceptions and sense of reality. Communication may differ based on who the sender is. In this model, if I, as a stranger, say "Good morning" to you, it has a slightly different meaning than if someone whom you have a deep affection for says "Good morning." Our lived experiences frame the communication.[2] From this model, we can appreciate the complex nature of communication and why developing strong communication skills is essential in professional development. **Figure 4.2** demonstrates the more complex interactional model of communication. Let's take communication one step further and explore the last model, transactional.[2]

The transactional model demonstrates the true complexities of communication. First, this model recognizes that the individuals are neither senders nor receivers; they simultaneously engage in a unique experience. Therefore, this model refers to the participants as communicators. The field of experience expands in this model, recognizing that although each communicator brings their own lived experiences, they also share the experience at the moment and that real-time shared interaction influences communication. Building on more communication dynamics, the transactional model recognizes

that communication is not simply the message and the feedback from that message but that communication consists of many messages stacked upon each other to influence the interaction. Wow! That simple "good morning" interaction just got far more complicated!

The transactional model allows for an understanding of how we frame our conversation and the opportunities and challenges in a single conversational exchange. Developing communication skills and understanding communication components gives health professionals the framework for successful conversations with patients, peers, and others.[2] **Figure 4.3** demonstrates the transactional communication model.

● COMPONENTS OF COMMUNICATION

Breaking down the communication models into their components is a valuable way to examine all the structural elements of communication. As humans, we use all our senses to process our interactions with the world. Communication is no exception. When communicating, we rely on our verbal capacity, ability to hear and listen, visual processing of nonverbal cues, and written communication. Even our sense of smell and taste can impact communication. Have you ever tried to pay attention to someone talking to you when there is a strong smell in the environment? Absolutely distracting! Reflecting on the transactional communication model, one can see how all of our senses play a role. Below, we define the key elements of communication and connect them to you as a professional.

Verbal – This is our most often-used mode of communication and probably one of the most important aspects of professionalism. Our persona is often defined by how we verbally communicate. Verbal communication can reflect knowledge, culture, background, and emotions within the message. Professional communication requires thoughtfulness before speaking and is tied to genuinely listening to the other parties involved. It requires appropriate word choices that reflect respect, clarity, and confidence yet are understandable to the receiver. Professional verbal delivery requires attention to tone,

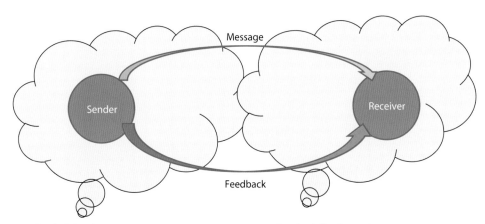

Sender's lived experiences   Receiver's lived experiences

FIGURE 4.2. Interactional Model of Communication.

CHAPTER 4 · Communication   **27**

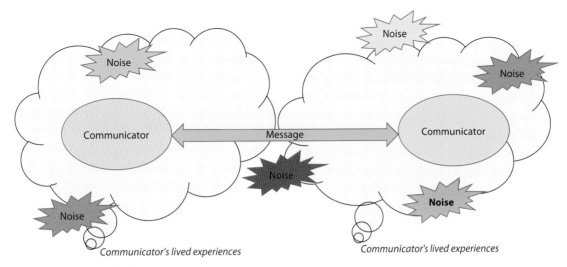

FIGURE 4.3. Transactional Model of Communication.

cadence, and awareness of nonverbal behaviors. Professional verbal communication implies understanding and integrating all messaging components and demonstrates the transactional model in action.[3]

Listening – This component is often overlooked. It is the means by which we gather information and gauge the situation: environment, emotions, and facts. Listening is required to truly understand, as it allows for focus on the situation, thoughtfulness in reaction, and leads to shared understanding. Listening requires patience, good eye contact, and the ability NOT to form a response as you are listening. Listening is an active skill that often requires practice. One must be willing to lean in and focus on what is being said. One must avoid looking for openings to insert opinions and defer judgment.[3]

Nonverbal – Nonverbal communication can take many forms. It can refer to written correspondence, but most often refers to the relay of a message through "body language"; position, distance, expressions, eye contact, and timing. Body language plays a crucial role in reinforcing or contradicting the verbal message and is reflected both in the speaking and listening mode.[3]

Written – Written messages now compose more of our communication modes than ever in formal and informal settings. Formal written communication can be seen in professional emails, correspondence, and medical documentation/record keeping. Informal means of written communication can be social email, texts, emojis, and social media. The key to appropriate written communication is knowledge of the receiver and the intent/nature of the communication. It is often best in professional communication to maintain formal relationships and standards of composition.

Environment – The physical environment in which communication occurs can influence the intended message. Simple things such as lighting, background noise, comfort, and seating arrangements can impact the conveyance of a message. For example, consider a discussion across a desk from a superior compared to the same conversation sitting next to a colleague. The former arrangement conveys more superiority or power structure which can often impact the process and outcome. The other conveys comfort and balance. Background noise levels can affect both sending and receiving information. It can impact the ability to listen, understand, and be understood. Speaking loudly over ambient sound can often change the tone and cadence of the delivery of the spoken word. Distractions and disruptions can derail any communication. Another consideration of the environment is the mood or atmosphere generated by others. High-stress emotions, such as anger and frustration, can be "felt," and this vibe can influence communication strategy and intent.[4] Think of the environment's influence on your body language, the ability to effectively deliver a message while simultaneously interpreting feedback, and your ability to be attentive to the conversation.

Experiences – We often do not consider how our personal experiences impact communication. Our previous encounters, emotions, education, roles, and situations can significantly influence how we send and receive messages. Previous personal experiences and situations may bias one toward an expectation of a positive or negative outcome. The way we impart messaging depends on the words we choose and the perceptions we create. Our level of education, verbal and written literacy, culture, and language can significantly transform our message to be perceived favorably or unfavorably. Similarly, these experiences influence our perceptions of the messaging received from others.

An astute professional can consider the relationship within the many communication components and adapt these complexities to attain shared understanding. **Table 4.1** summarizes key points for each element of communication.

Reflection Moment

Think about some recent conversations and communications you had recently. Consider the experiences you brought to the discussion, the experiences of the other individuals, the

TABLE 4.1. Elements of Communication

Communication	Examples	Considerations
Verbal	Face-to-face Telephone Group discussions Presentations	Unique styles of communication Behavioral style
Listening	Reflective Distracted	Use empathy to improve interaction.
Nonverbal Body Language	Body Language Sign Language	Provide nonverbal cues and understand nonverbal cues.
Written	Formal: Emails, medical records documentation, correspondence Informal: text, signs, and symbols	Understand your audience. Consider the nature of the subject matter.
Environment	Lighting Noise Comfort Seating arrangements Distractions Atmosphere Smells	Be attentive to the surrounding area in terms of concrete and perceptual context. Redirect the conversation if the environment has too much distraction for the participants.
Experiences	Previous interactions Emotions Education Culture Role Biases	Be open-minded with others. Understand how our lived experiences can impact perception.

environment you shared, and how the messages built upon one another.

1. What communication interaction had a positive outcome?
2. What communication interaction had a negative outcome?
3. What factors from the list above influenced those positive and negative outcomes?
4. What components of the model might you consider differently in the future to move potentially adverse outcomes to positive outcomes?

● ASSESSING COMMUNICATION

So far, this chapter has built a foundation for understanding professional communication by examining communication models and their components. Additionally, other helpful tools provide professionals with an even deeper understanding of how individuals communicate. These tools give you a way to predict how interactions may play out with different individuals, giving you strategies to modify your communication to promote a better outcome. An example of one of these tools is the DISC Behavioral Style Assessment.

The DISC Behavioral Assessment is a valid and reliable assessment that quantifies human behaviors into four quadrants. DISC is an acronym that stands for four leading personality profiles: (D) dominance, (I) influence, (S) steadiness, and (C) conscientiousness. The theoretical work of William Marston, a physiological psychologist with a Ph.D. from Harvard, as published in "*Emotions of Normal People*" (1928),

provided the foundation for the current DISC behavioral styles tool. Marston's original work was used to develop the DISC assessment, which is helpful in examining working relationships and team interactions. In addition, this vital tool can help you understand the communication patterns of different people.[4]

So, what exactly does DISC mean? The DISC indicates that people are different but predictably different.[4] Why does this matter when we are talking about communication? Well, to start, we discussed above in the models of communication that communication is a complex interaction, so having some way to organize components of communication is helpful. This is what a tool like DISC provides us. The DISC Behavioral Assessment gives us clues as to how different people communicate. Right now, you are thinking…so what! I am not going to perform this behavioral assessment on each person. Of course not! However, we can look for clues about a person's behavioral style through verbal and nonverbal communication. In doing so, we can adapt our communications to fit their style best. This is important because people respond best when they receive information in a manner that they relate to. It's often referred to as the "Platinum Rule." The Platinum Rule states that we should interact with people how they prefer. It provides for a more thoughtful approach to dealing with others. The DISC behavioral style is a tool that helps us accomplish the Platinum Rule.

Finally, one convenient aspect of the DISC behavioral style tool exists. Nearly 65% of individuals have "Steadiness" as their primary behavioral style. This implies that if you start by

TABLE 4.2. DISC Profile

Style	Population % with Primary Style	Verbal Communication	Non-verbal Communication	Words and Phrases to Use	Words and Phrases and Words to Avoid
D-Dominant	3-5%	Direct communicator, very little patience for small talk, often loud and forceful communicator, will interrupt others	High use of gestures and a lot of hand movement when communicating	Advantage Decisive Quick Efficient	Patience Inconsistent Follow directions
I-Influence	10-15%	A great deal of tone variation in their voice, enjoys long conversations; enjoy long explanations but are poor listeners and will often lose interest when others are talking	High use of gestures and facial expressions	Flexible Inspiring Exciting	Ordinary Quiet Strict Routine
S-Steadiness	55-65%	Warm discussions, often soft-spoken, great listeners	Small hand gestures when talking	Consistent Usual Secure	Unexpected Urgent Confrontation
C-Compliant	10-15%	Very direct and to the point, will ask for clarification of what someone is saying	Very reserved with minimal to no hand gestures	Proven Precise Verified	Educated guess Experimental Imagine

Adapted from Bonnstetter & Suiter[4]

understanding the "Steadiness" style and providing communication that aligns with their behavioral style, you will be on the right track with most people! **Table 4.2** below outlines the four behavioral styles and how each communicates verbally and nonverbally. The table also provides words and phrases that work to consider with each style.[4]

After reviewing the table, take a moment and think about the people in your life. Which individuals fit these characteristics? For example, do you know someone who always tells fun stories and wants to connect with many people? If so, that person probably enjoys communicating with the "Influencing" behavioral style. Likewise, people in your life who communicate more softly, are good listeners and enjoy discussion with close friends probably employ the "Steadiness" behavior style. By considering these four behavioral styles when you interact with others and practicing how to communicate differently based on the other person's behavioral style, you gain a valuable strategy for effective communication that works in all situations and with everyone. It's truly that powerful! If you want to explore more about DISC behavioral styles or complete a DISC Behavioral Style assessment for yourself, there is a list of useful websites and references at the end of this chapter.

The models and components of communication and ways to assess individual communication styles all provide a foundation for you to consider how communication plays into your professional development. However, to fully appreciate your communication expectations as a professional, it is important to add the framework from guiding documents to your working communication foundation.

● PROFESSIONAL COMMUNICATION

The overall goal of communication is to create shared understanding. An effective communicator responds in a manner that incorporates the perspective of others. Therefore, effective communication is a critical element of professional development and an expectation in health care. *Professional Behaviors for the 21st Century* points explicitly to communication as a key component of professionalism for physical therapy professionals. This document provides a valuable resource by defining and clarifying skills that guide the progression of communication skills throughout one's career. Refer to **Table 4.3** for expectations of effective communication at varying timeframes in our professional journey.

Physical therapy professionals need effective communication to ensure successful patient/client outcomes and positive interactions with their peers, business associates, and the community. Pulling together the models, components, and assessment and guidance documents provides the foundation for building skills as an effective communicator. Let's take some time to apply these skills to case studies and explore how communication develops from an emerging to reflecting and, finally, to an influencing clinician. The following section provides an example and three additional case studies for you to apply your foundational knowledge.

● CASE STUDIES

This section explores four case studies focusing on (1) patient/client interaction, (2) peer interaction, (3) business associate interaction, and (4) community interaction. Each case study considers how the emerging, reflecting, and influencing professional communicates.

TABLE 4.3. Guidance for Professional Communication for Physical Therapist and Physical Therapist Assistants[5]

Core Documents	Definitions	Skills
Professional Behaviors for the 21st Century	The ability to communicate effectively (i.e., verbal, nonverbal, reading, writing, and listening) for varied audiences and purposes.	**Beginning Level:** Demonstrates understanding of the English language (verbal and written): uses correct grammar, accurate spelling and expression, legible handwriting. Recognizes the impact of nonverbal communication on self and others. Recognizes the verbal and nonverbal characteristics that portray confidence. Utilizes electronic communication appropriately. **Intermediate Level:** Utilizes and modifies communication (verbal, nonverbal, written, and electronic) to meet the needs of different audiences. Restates, reflects, and clarifies message(s). Communicates collaboratively with both individuals and groups. Collects necessary information from all pertinent individuals in the patient/client management process. Provides effective education (verbal, nonverbal, written, and electronic). **Entry Level:** Demonstrates the ability to maintain appropriate control of the communication exchange with individuals and groups. Presents persuasive and explanatory verbal, written, or electronic messages with logical organization and sequencing. Maintains open and constructive communication. Utilizes communication technology effectively and efficiently. **Post Entry Level:** Adapts messages to address needs, expectations, and prior knowledge of the audience to maximize learning. Effectively delivers messages capable of influencing patients, the community, and society. Provides education locally, regionally, and/or nationally. Mediates conflict.

Adapted with permission from May W, Kontney L, Iglarsh A. Professional behaviors for the 21st Century. Marquette University; 2010.

CASE STUDY 1
Patient/Client—I understand those instructions

Payton is a Physical Therapist working in an outpatient center connected with the local health care system. They graduated from a Doctor of Physical Therapy program six years ago. Payton enjoys the high-paced atmosphere of the outpatient center and its diverse caseload. Payton is scheduled to evaluate a new patient, George. George is a 74-year-old man who fell off his ladder while cleaning out the gutters on his home approximately two months ago. He sustained several injuries during his fall, including fractures to his right arm and right leg. George has used a wheelchair for mobility since his fall and is now cleared to begin therapy to include exercise and ambulation activities.

Payton meets George in his wheelchair in the middle of the gym because all the private exam rooms are currently occupied. He is staring down at his lap and appears disinterested in most activities around him. His wife, Julia, is seated in a chair next to him. She is chatting with one of the patients exercising on the mat table next to her. Occasionally, Julia turns back to George and asks him if he is OK. When he nods accordingly, she returns to the conversation without skipping a beat.

Payton has a hectic day scheduled and has only 45 minutes to complete the initial evaluation for George. They know they must gather the necessary clinical data and

provide instructions for a home exercise program during this session. As Payton reviews the notes provided by the home health therapist who recently discharged George, they see that George often demonstrated poor safety and difficulty with his current weight-bearing limitations. He was occasionally confused and relied heavily on his wife to reinforce instructions. As Payton approaches George, he appears nervous and looks to his wife for support. **Table 4.4** outlines the communication components of this scenario.

 EMERGING PROFESSIONAL

As an emerging professional, Payton demonstrates an awareness of the challenges present in this scenario, including the less-than-ideal environment, tight time constraints, and the differences in each individual's communication preferences. However, Payton does not consider significant modifications to any factors to place the interaction in an ideal situation. As an emerging professional, Payton stays focused on collecting pertinent information regarding the individual's clinical presentation. However, they may miss the cues from both George and Julia regarding their unique communication needs. Payton relies heavily on Julia for information as she is more verbal. The interaction produces an effective result of data collection

TABLE 4.4. Case Study 1—Communication Components

Components	Payton	George	Julia
Verbal	Payton is often direct and to the point and does not enjoy small talk.	George is soft-spoken and prefers a slow, detailed conversation.	Julia loves the art of talking. She tells stories and jokes often.
Listening	Because they like to stay on schedule, Payton is often challenged to listen to a complete story from others, especially if it contains many details. As a result, Payton often interrupts to redirect to the task at hand.	George has always been a great listener. He prefers to listen rather than speak. But lately, he has found listening more challenging, which is frustrating.	Julia listens long enough to find a point that connects to a story she wants to tell.
Non-verbal	Payton talks with their hands and uses big gestures.	George keeps his hands in his lap, avoids eye contact, and uses small gestures.	Julia uses lots of hand and facial gestures.
Written	Peyton prefers concise communication, often with bullet points. Writing is not something Payton enjoys.	George enjoyed writing and would still write his wife long love letters after 50 years of marriage. However, recently he has been unable to write due to his injury.	Julia also enjoys writing and will send long emails and letters to friends and family.
Experience	Payton is from the millennial generation, an athlete in college, and loves to exercise. They enjoy patients they can push and strive to use creativity in their programs.	George is a retired factory worker with a high school diploma. He worked at the same location and lived in the same house his entire adult life. He prefers to vacation with their children and grandchildren at the same lake every year. His hobbies are fishing and hiking.	Julia is a Certified Nursing Assistant although, recently, she has placed work on hold to take care of George. Julia loves to travel and explore and often goes on trips with friends. She belongs to several different community clubs and volunteers her time often as one of the club officers. All of this activity is currently on hold since George's injury.
Behavioral Style	Payton demonstrates a primary "Dominant" style.	George demonstrates a primary "Steadiness" style.	Julia demonstrates a primary "Influencing" style.
Environment	The environment is a noisy outpatient gym with many people and distractions. The setting may contain uncomfortable aspects, such as other individuals' injuries or disabilities. There is no privacy for George and Julia.		

and a relevant home exercise program. However, George may feel unheard and have several unanswered questions. Payton may take several more visits to measure George's comprehension of their interactions and gain his trust and full engagement.

 REFLECTING PROFESSIONAL

As a reflecting professional, Payton realizes the challenges created by the environment and picks up on the communication styles of both George and Julia within the first few moments of their interaction. As a reflective professional, Payton knows how to accommodate George and Julia by finding a better location for the evaluation, slowing down the evaluation process, and putting their goals and plans aside to make George and Julia more comfortable. Payton realizes that they need to listen intently to George and redirect Julia to create a better interaction with George. In this scenario, Payton realizes that an evaluation for George will take more than one session to complete and allows the necessary time to explain the process. Payton encourages questions, asks open-ended questions in turn, and works to engage George in much of the conversation. By the end of the appointment, Payton builds the foundation

of a trusting relationship with George and engages and demonstrates appreciation for Julia's efforts in his care. The couple leaves the appointment feeling heard and appreciated but still unclear on some critical process components.

 INFLUENCING PROFESSIONAL

As an influencing professional, Payton immediately notes the potential challenges of the situation before even interacting with George and Julia. They thoroughly observe the environment and connect the observations with challenges stated by the home health clinician in the medical record. Payton redirects their client load by assigning tasks to support personnel allowing for more time for the evaluation with George. Payton also finds a quiet place location, and after a warm and sincere greeting, they move George and Julia personally. Payton listens intently to Julia's most recent story acknowledging highlights of it with warm facial expressions and brief comments. During the evaluation, Payton asks open-ended questions of George but does not disregard Julia's need to interject stories supporting George's answers. Payton skillfully intermingles clinical evaluation activities with warm conversation while staying focused on the session's goals. Payton recognizes the key instructions that George requires for safety and spends time reviewing them with George asking for clarification in a "teach-back" method in which Payton asks both George and Julia to state what each understood about the instructions in their own words. By the session's end, George and Julia feel supported and understood. They tell Payton they understand the path to recovery and what they must do to get George back on his feet.

CASE STUDY 2

Peer—You are not listening to me. Why do you have to be so difficult?

Sam and Dwight are the only two physical therapists employed in a home health company. They both started working for the company about five years ago. Sam and Dwight have a collegial relationship; however, they do not collaborate regarding patients or work as a team. Sam has more seniority, but Dwight works more hours to cover weekends. The company is growing and has recently hired a physical therapist assistant (PTA) to help manage the growing caseload. Before hiring the PTA, Sam and Dwight could control their caseloads and did not have to coordinate schedules with anyone else except for occasional vacation coverage. As a result, both enjoyed their autonomy and preferred to do their own thing.

The company decides that the PTA will assist one of the therapists and needs to determine who will provide supervision. The designated supervisor will receive a small monthly stipend for the extra workload. Sam feels he should supervise the PTA since he has more seniority. On the other hand, Dwight thinks that since he is the therapist who always volunteers to take extra evaluations on the weekend, he could best utilize the help of the PTA.

The therapy supervisor brings both Sam and Dwight into the office for a meeting to make a plan for the newly hired PTA. The therapy supervisor lays out the coverage territory and initiates the discussion. **Table 4.5** considers the communication components of this case study.

Sam is represented as the emerging and reflecting professional below. As a practice exercise, consider Sam's characteristics as an influencing professional.

 EMERGING PROFESSIONAL

As an emerging professional, Sam demonstrates awareness of his challenges in communicating with Dwight and the supervisor in this scenario. Although Sam realizes that the lack of face-to-face interaction with Dwight and their brevity in communication may make discussing this new scenario more difficult, he finds considering other forms of interaction challenging. For example, during the conversation, Sam does not control his hand gestures or his facial expressions as he tries to support his case.

Sam works to "win" the discussion and does not realize the long-term impact of going into a conversation to win. He sees the small stipend as an advantage since he has not received a pay rate increase in the past year. He fails to listen attentively as he interjects his points, and his facial and hand expressions denote frustration with the situation. As a result, Sam misses the opportunity to gain insight into the value of the new team member for the company and the impact on the weekend work schedule.

 REFLECTING PROFESSIONAL

As a reflecting professional, Sam understands the need to listen first to gain the facts regarding the situation. Therefore, he maintains a neutral expression as he listens to

Component	Sam and Dwight
TABLE 4.5. Case Study 2—Communication Components	
Verbal	Both are often direct in their communication and feel that friendly discussions and small talk are for after work.
Listening	Both listen only to find the necessary data to answer their questions. As experienced home health clinicians, they value their time and want facts only.
Nonverbal	Both use large hand gestures and express emotion with facial gestures.
Written	Both prefer brief bulleted points and concise information. They often do not reply to emails if they feel they are unnecessary.
Experience	Both love the autonomy of home health. This clinical setting provides them with personal freedom and the ability to make expert decisions independently. In addition, they both enjoy flexible schedules that allow them to do other things.
Behavioral Style	Both demonstrate a primary "Dominance" behavioral style.
Environment	The home health environment is an autonomous clinical environment that allows clinicians flexibility. Adding a PTA to this environment will aid in productivity but reduce some autonomy by decreasing the flexibility of scheduling and increasing the workload for oversight of the PTA and patient management. The meeting at the office is held in a small conference room at the end of the day.

the supervisor explain the situation and to Dwight as he presents his challenges with the weekend work. In doing so, Sam learns the reason for hiring the PTA and the potential upside benefits to the company. In addition, Sam hears about the company's growth and the potential for additional leadership positions. Sam also learns that the PTA resides in an area closer to Dwight's treatment territory. Sam gains valuable information that allows him to move the conversation forward for a more productive outcome by listening first to understand and placing his natural desire to win the conversation to the side.

 INFLUENCING PROFESSIONAL

How should Sam approach this as an influencing professional? Consider the following questions:

1. How should Sam prepare for this meeting?
2. What experiences might he bring to the meeting?
3. How would he use listening and nonverbal skills in this situation?
4. Can you recommend any verbal, nonverbal, environmental, or behavioral changes that might impact the outcome of this meeting?

CASE STUDY 3
Business Associate—This team is not getting anywhere

The director of an inpatient rehabilitation hospital recently assigned Michaeline, a physical therapist (PT), Yolanda, an occupational therapist (OT), and Rachelle, a speech-language pathologist (SLP) to work collaboratively on developing a new clinical pathway for patients diagnosed with Parkinson's disease. Michaeline is a recent graduate of a clinical neuroscience residency that she completed immediately following graduation from her Doctor of Physical Therapy program. Yolanda has over ten years of clinical experience, primarily working with children in the school system but has focused on adult rehab in the past year. Rachelle is the lead therapist for the SLP program's neuro team.

The three individuals meet via video conference since each works different hours in different departments. The video conference meeting style allows flexibility without significantly impacting everyone's schedule. The first few meetings get off to a challenging start with some technical issues and interruptions. The team decides to break up some of the research and development of the program to work more efficiently. Each team member shares their findings and suggestions when they return to the next call. Michaeline starts by reviewing several pages of in-depth research regarding the historical overview of clinical pathways and concludes with a proposal that they conduct a pilot trial of several different methods before moving forward. Yolanda is lost halfway through Michaeline's explanation. She repeatedly interrupts Michaeline during her review to express her feelings about the information. She suggests they should choose a clinical pathway and see if everyone else on the rehabilitation team thinks it is a good idea. Finally,

Rachelle, who believes she should lead the way since she is already a team leader of a neuro SLP program, has outlined a pathway that she believes will lead to the most efficient and effective method. She thanks Michaeline and Yolanda for their work on the project but, after listening to their input, believes that she will take her pathway to the dIrector as the decision from the group. Both Michaeline and Yolanda are highly frustrated. Michaeline believes that Rachelle is not expressing respect for research and wants to do things based on her personal experience. Yolanda feels that Rachelle communicated in a controlling manner and didn't consider the information shared by herself and Michaeline. As the meeting time on the teleconference runs out, they end their conversation. They all feel frustrated and have not made a decision. Two weeks later, when the director meets to hear their results, there is no progress to report, and each expresses their frustration. While this project has gone off the rails, it allows the team to learn from each other and gain valuable communication insights. **Table 4.6** outlines the communication components of this case study.

Michaeline is reflected as an emerging professional below. First, consider Michaeline's characteristics as a reflecting and influencing professional as a practice exercise. Then consider Yolanda and Rachelle's communication at each level.

 EMERGING PROFESSIONAL

As an emerging professional, Michaeline focuses on improving her knowledge and demonstrating her expertise. She is cautious about discussing clinical aspects from the perspective of her personal experience and prefers to use others' experiences in the form of research and case studies. She is unsure how to best share her ideas with the more verbal Yolanda and Rachelle. After sharing her research and a detailed plan, she faces resistance and a lack of agreement. She is unsure how to proceed next, so she becomes quiet and does not speak up throughout the meeting.

The video conference interaction is challenging for Michaeline as she finds it difficult to insert her voice and read the others on the team. In addition, because both Yolanda and Rachelle are more dynamic in gestures and facial expressions, Michaeline is intimidated and backs away from the conversation.

Michaeline leaves the conversation frustrated by the perceived lack of desire of the other two for the best evidence-based clinical pathway. She considers their lack of focus on the details an issue with "seasoned clinicians" who rely solely on their experiences, not evidence. As a result, Michaeline develops a sense that the project will not represent the best evidence-based approach.

 REFLECTING PROFESSIONAL

Questions to consider:

How might Michaeline use a blend of experiential clinical knowledge with evidence-based research to communicate in this scenario?

TABLE 4.6. Case Study 3—Communication Components

Component	Michaeline	Yolanda	Rachelle
Verbal	Michaeline is quiet and tends to wait to discuss items until she knows her facts. She does not appreciate small talk.	Yolanda loves to tell stories. She tends to talk a lot and often interrupts others, so she doesn't forget to share her ideas.	Rachelle is often direct in her communication and feels that friendly discussions and small talk are something for after work.
Listening	Michaeline's quiet nature and shyness often come across as not listening. She strives to listen to every detail but becomes frustrated when someone is not concise and adds detail without a specific reason.	Yolanda listens to find the next spot to add to the conversation. She enjoys talking and often gets excited about how she can add to what someone is saying.	Rachelle listens well when she feels it is essential to listen, such as a patient history; however, when she thinks that individuals are talking too much or slowing down a process, she easily blocks them out because she already has an answer.
Nonverbal	Michaeline uses very few hand or facial gestures while talking.	Yolanda uses excessive facial and hand gestures while speaking and listening to others. Her facial gestures can lead to distraction for others when they are talking.	Rachelle uses large hand gestures and will use facial gestures when she believes it will give her the advantage to get her point across.
Written	Michaeline writes in detail to ensure exactness and provide supporting evidence. In addition, she always attaches supporting evidence to emails so that others can also examine the data.	Yolanda prefers to share information verbally and usually does not write things down because of her outstanding memory. As a result, she struggles with clinical documentation and often has to clarify documentation.	Rachelle prefers brief bulleted points. Therefore, her written communications contain the necessary information only.
Experience	Michaeline's career focus is on becoming a respected expert in the field of neurology. She is accomplishing this through additional schooling, research, and continued evidence-based practice.	Yolanda is trying to fit in with her new clinical team. Although comfortable in her pediatric role for the last ten years, she finds it hard to make friends and have the same level of fun in this new role.	Rachelle's career focus is moving from clinical care to administration, and she sees these collaborative activities as a means to achieve her goals and as a way to demonstrate her ability to take charge of the situation.
Behavioral Style	Michaeline demonstrates a primary "Compliance" behavioral style.	Yolanda demonstrates a primary "Influencing" behavioral style.	Rachelle demonstrates a primary "Dominance" behavioral style.
Environment	The environment is a remote video meeting filled with distractions with the ability to mute and turn off the video feed. There is a time constraint on the call. The team does not work together regularly; this is the first time they have done a project together.		

1. How might Michaeline use her awareness of the behavioral styles of others when sharing her research?
2. What strategies might Michaeline employ to ensure her voice is heard during a video conference call?

 INFLUENCING PROFESSIONAL

Questions to consider:

1. How might Michaeline prepare the other two clinicians for a more engaging conversation focused on the essential aspects of evidence-based research around this topic?
2. What strategies might Michaeline learn to redirect Yolanda when she interrupts or to refocus Rachelle when she loses interest in the details?
3. How might Michaeline express her ideas to others during a video conference to ensure that everyone engages in the conversations in a meaningful manner?

CASE STUDY 4

Community Interaction—Let me tell you about our clinic

Arifa is a clinical director for a private practice pediatric clinic that employs five therapists. The clinic owner just announced the sale of the practice to a large competitor in the area. The owner told Arifa that this is an excellent opportunity to demonstrate their clinical practice knowledge and present their case for the growth of this pediatric clinic within the new company. Although Arifa feels very comfortable leading the small team, most of their experience is clinical, and rarely have they presented to other professionals. The presentation is in one week, and Arifa will have 30 minutes to provide an overview of the team, their accomplishments, and Arifa's vision for the future. **Table 4.7** describes Arifa's communication attributes.

As a practice exercise, consider Arifa's characteristics as an emerging, reflecting, and influencing professional and how they might impact her presentation.

TABLE 4.7. Case Study 4—Arifa's Communication Attributes

Component	Arifa
Verbal	Arifa is usually soft-spoken and enjoys long conversations in a one-on-one environment. They like to talk through things and will call each team member individually to get their input.
Listening	Arifa is a great listener, sometimes listens too long, does not redirect others, and therefore gives too much personal time.
Nonverbal	Arifa uses small hand gestures and warm facial expressions.
Written	Arifa writes long emails and uses detail to describe clinical scenarios.
Experience	Arifa has seven years of clinical experience. In addition, Arifa has been the clinical director for two years.
Behavioral Style	Arifa demonstrates the primary "Steadiness" behavioral style.
Environment	The presentation is in a small conference room with six leaders from the acquiring organization. All of the team members have business backgrounds. The company's owner presents first and introduces Arifa to provide an overview of their role and vision for the program.

 EMERGING PROFESSIONAL

Questions to consider:

1. What skills might Arifa need to complete this project?
2. What barriers might Arifa face as an emerging professional?
3. How might this experience help Arifa grow as a professional?

 REFLECTING PROFESSIONAL

Questions to consider:

1. What resources and experiences might Arifa draw on as a reflecting professional?
2. What barriers might Arifa face as she communicates with others?
3. How might this experience help Arifa move toward becoming an influencing professional?

 INFLUENCING PROFESSIONAL

Questions to consider:

1. What resources and experiences might Arifa draw on as an influencing professional?
2. How might Arifa frame this presentation to meet the behavioral styles of others?
3. How might Arifa use this experience to engage emerging and reflective professionals on their team?

It's time to put the knowledge you gained from examining the models, components, and assessment of professional communication and putting them into practice in the case studies to use in your professional development.

● PERSONAL DEVELOPMENT: COMMUNICATION

Take a moment to reflect on your communication with patients/clients and your peers in one-on-one interactions, as a team member, and within the community in which your profession engages.

Reflection Moment

Consider the following questions:

1. What specific elements are you attentive to when communicating with others?
2. What DISC behavioral style do you most relate to and why?
3. In what communication environments are you most confident, and in which do you lack confidence?

After reflecting on these areas, complete the table below. Do you consider yourself an emerging, reflecting, or influencing professional regarding your communication? Complete your current communication skill level in **Table 4.8**.

Use the answers from Table 4.8 to complete your professional development plan for communication in **Table 4.9**. Based on where you are now, what areas need development to ensure growth in professional communication? Remember, completing the plan in each chapter helps build your overall professional development plan at the end of the book.

TABLE 4.8. Current Level of Communication Skills

My Current Level of Development	
How do you prefer to interact verbally?	
How well do you listen?	
Are you aware of nonverbal interaction characteristics?	
Written communication preferences	
Are you aware of your experiences with communication?	
Are you aware of the environment of communication?	

TABLE 4.9. Professional Development Plan for Communication

Communication Goals (No More Than 2-3)	Tactics to Accomplish My Communication Goals	The Measure of Success for My Communication Goals	Accountability Partner: Who Will I Share My Goals with, and How Will I Check In with Them

References

1. Leonard P. Exploring ways to manage healthcare professional-patient communication issues. *Support Care Cancer.* 2017;25:7-9. doi:10.1007/s00520-017-3635-6.

2. Pierce T. *The Evolution of Human Communication: From Theory to Practice.* 2nd ed. Pressbooks; 2019. https://ecampusontario.pressbooks.pub/evolutionhumancommunication/chapter/the-evolution-of-human-communication/.

3. Mueller K. *Communication from the inside Out.* McGraw Hill; 2010. https://fadavispt.mhmedical.com/content.aspx?bookid=1887&sectionid=147151197. Accessed May 8, 2021.

4. Bonnstetter B, Suiter J. *The Universal Language DISC Reference Manual.* Target Training International; 1984.

5. May W, Kontney L, Iglarsh A. Professional behaviors for the 21st century. Published online 2010. https://www.marquette.edu/physical-therapy/documents/professional-behaviors.pdf.

chapter 5

Emotional Intelligence

Although we often do not realize it, emotions play a significant role in all aspects of our life. From our daily interactions to essential decisions, emotions influence our actions, thoughts, and relationships with others. In health care, emotions can have life-altering effects on patients and health care providers. An awareness of the role of emotions in our lives and appropriate strategies to manage emotions within our interactions are necessary tools in health care delivery. In this chapter, we examine the components of emotional intelligence and discuss ways to develop skills and strategies for the application of emotional intelligence in our personal and professional interactions.

● EMOTIONS: OUR BRAINS AND BODIES

Our feelings make us uniquely human, and it's important to consider how our body processes and uses emotions. As humans, our emotions are built into every action. Physiologically, our brains are wired to leverage the power of emotions before our rational thoughts. **Figure 5.1** briefly illustrates the pathways of emotional and rational thinking. As you can see, a signal enters the brain and is initially sent through the thalamus to the amygdala for emotional processing and the neocortex for

rational processing. The emotional pathway is smaller, making it just milliseconds faster than the rational thought pathway. This smaller and faster pathway often allows emotions to influence our responses before rational thought can intervene. Next time you hear someone say, "Don't be so emotional," well, in fact, we are all wired to be so emotional!

In our day-to-day life, the initial emotional response can be beneficial. For example, if we see a harmful object, we become fearful. This emotion, in turn, triggers our flight or fight response which is very helpful if we need to run from that harmful object. Rationally, we may then realize that no harm will come to us, and we don't have to run, but it is still in our best interest to be prepared. Our emotions often serve as a trigger for the body's protection.

Although the initial emotional response may be helpful, there are many times when it gets us in trouble, and we regret acting on that early emotional response. Consider this scenario, a family member leaves their things on the floor in the hallway, and you trip over them. This makes you angry and you instantly begin lecturing them about being irresponsible. You do this before you realize they are upset and left their items in the hallway when they received a troubling phone call. Here, rational

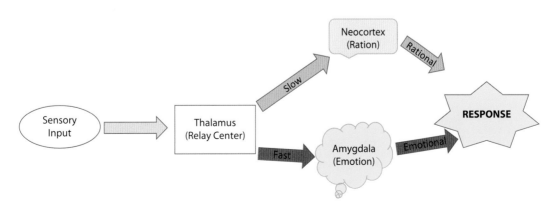

FIGURE 5.1. Emotional and Rational Thought Pathway.

observation of the situation may have changed the response to tripping over the items and could have saved some distress for a loved one. This is an example of how emotional intelligence comes into play. If one has strategies to recognize and regulate heightened emotions quickly, it allows the opportunity to use rational thinking and apply techniques, such as empathy, to interactions with others. Let's look at the definition of emotional intelligence and break it down into its components.[1]

DEFINING EMOTIONAL INTELLIGENCE

To define emotional intelligence best, it is necessary first to explain the concept of intelligence and explore how the theories of different types of intelligence evolved. As the study of the human mind and how we learn grew, so did the definition of intelligence. A working definition of intelligence is "the ability to learn, to reason well, to solve novel problems, and deal effectively with challenges, often unpredictable, that one confronts in daily life."[2] In the 1920s, a psychologist named Edward L. Thorndike introduced the idea that there was more than one type of intelligence. Thorndike proposed three types of intelligence: abstract, mechanical, and social intelligence. He defined social intelligence as "the ability to get along with people in general, ease in society, knowledge of social matters, and the insight into the personalities and moods of strangers." This concept was the foundational theory for the future development of emotional intelligence.[2,3] Although the idea that social intelligence plays a vital role existed throughout the 1900s, it was largely ignored as an essential aspect of intelligence worthy of testing and evaluation. In fact, in 1940, when David Wechsler, a Romanian-American psychologist and researcher in the area of intelligence, suggested including social intelligence as a component of Intelligence Quotient (IQ) testing, his suggestion was not acknowledged. Therefore, IQ testing, which became a foundational evaluation of intelligence for many decades to come, completely ignores social intelligence. It wasn't until the 1980s that scientists explored the concept of multiple intelligence types again. In his work, Howard Gardner, a developmental psychologist, described eight types of intelligence, including interpersonal and intrapersonal intelligence. The actual idea of emotional intelligence is relatively new and did not appear in the literature until the 1990s when Peter Salovey and John D. Mayer published their article entitled "Emotional Intelligence" in the Journal of *Imagination, Cognition, and Personality*.[3] These psychologists defined emotional intelligence as " the ability to perceive accurately, appraise and express emotions, the ability to access and/or generate feelings when they facilitate thought; the ability to understand emotion and emotional knowledge; and the ability to regulate emotions to promote emotional and intellectual growth."[1]

Although comprehensive, Salovey and Mayer's definition may lead to more questions than answers about emotional intelligence. So, let's take a few moments to break this concept into a few more manageable components that we will explore in more detail throughout this chapter. First and foremost, it is essential to understand that emotional intelligence is a learned behavior. This is great news because it means that you can apply strategies to build your emotional intelligence and measure how it improves over time. As physical therapy practitioners, this fits nicely with our professional focus on setting measurable and obtainable goals and plans. Second, emotional intelligence breaks down into smaller pieces that act as building blocks for each other. This means you don't have to jump into developing emotional intelligence skills in all aspects of your life simultaneously. Instead, it allows you to choose small manageable components of emotional intelligence to work on to build a foundation for future skills. Finally, the elements of emotional intelligence consist of examination of yourself and your emotions and then extending outward to apply these skills toward others.

EMOTIONAL INTELLIGENCE: WHY IT MATTERS SO MUCH IN HEALTH CARE

Before we dive into the nuts and bolts of building emotional intelligence, it is important to understand its impact on health care. This section briefly describes the literature supporting emotional intelligence in health care and how these skills evolved to play an important role in entry-level education and life-long learning of health care providers.

Studies examining emotional intelligence's influence in the workforce point to its role in successful careers. For example, emotional intelligence has been shown to impact job performance significantly. Statistics show that 90% of high-performing employees demonstrate a high degree of emotional intelligence, and more than 50% of job performance satisfaction is linked to high emotional intelligence. In fact, studies find that people with high emotional intelligence scores earn an average of $29,000 more per year than counterparts with lower emotional intelligence scores.[1]

Studies examining the relationship of emotional intelligence as it relates to patient safety and outcomes demonstrate the connection between the emotional intelligence of health care providers and the quality of care. As an example, research connects emotional intelligence to better nursing performance and improved patient safety. In the field of occupational therapy, the ability to predict and manage others' emotions is linked to improved clinical performance.[4] In other studies on the emotional intelligence of physicians, researchers found that physicians with lower social-emotional intelligence skills were sued more often.[3] When examining the perceived stress of students in a variety of medical professions, those with higher emotional intelligence had a lower level of perceived stress throughout their education.[3] A growing body of research supports the positive relationship of emotional intelligence in health care. Consider a career such as physical therapy, where the majority of your day requires your ability to regulate your emotional response and connect with others. With an understanding and awareness of emotional intelligence, you have the opportunity to improve your well-being, impact your career, and improve your interactions with peers and patients. Now let's examine the components of emotional intelligence.

COMPONENTS OF EMOTIONAL INTELLIGENCE

Emotional intelligence requires you to understand and regulate your emotions and be motivated to stay focused on tasks at hand, even when emotions are heightened. Once you understand the components of personal emotional intelligence, you can begin to examine your ability to discern the emotions of others, use strategies to understand the emotional regulation of those around you and expand your ability to support others. This next section explores the areas of personal and social emotional intelligence and provides examples and strategies for professional growth and development.

Personal Components

One way to consider emotional intelligence is to use the analogy of temperature. Temperature is most pleasant at moderate levels. Emotions are the same; they are most tolerable when not overly hot or cold. For example, anger, frustration, excitement, indifference, or apathy may challenge our ability to engage with the world. You want to consider taking your emotional temperature when thinking about your emotions. This is the first step of self-awareness and is required to begin using self-regulation and motivation skills.

Self-awareness – This first step of emotional intelligence, self-awareness, often seems like something that is just apparent. You may think, "Of course, I am aware of my emotions!" But are you really aware of them most of the time? Or are there times when emotions go unnoticed until they influence a decision or an action and, on later reflection, you realize that your emotions made a significant impact on the outcome? Consider this scenario: You are upset with a coworker and say something out of frustration in a staff meeting. The second you say it, you regret the action. Can you identify with this scenario? If you have ever done this or something similar… you just forgot to leverage your emotional intelligence. This action exemplifies how our emotions get the best of us and drive our reactions. Emotional intelligence skills allow you to be more aware of these moments and learn ways that bring that emotional temperature from "red-hot" or "icy-cold" back to a moderate temperature that allows the neocortex and more rational thought to drive actions.

Let's consider some helpful practices to grow the self-awareness component of emotional intelligence. First, make a conscious effort throughout the day to pause and ask yourself: What is my emotional state right now? What is my temperature? What things in my life are affecting my emotional temperature? Just asking these simple questions and reflecting on your emotional state throughout the day can help you to become more aware of your emotions. To take this to the next level of emotional intelligence, consider keeping track of your daily emotions and things that trigger these emotions in a journal or the notes section of your phone. By having this log, you can see patterns and better understand the what, who, when, and where of your emotions and triggers. For example, you might start to see that a coworker always picks up your spirits, you become more frustrated at a certain time of day, or you always feel peaceful when you get to your yoga class. Knowing these ebbs and flows gives you insight into your emotions, and you can then move to the next step of self-regulation.

Self-regulation – Self-regulation is useful in our day-to-day lives and a powerful tool when working in the highly dynamic health care field. Self-regulation strategies allow you to return your emotional state to a moderate temperature. Sometimes you learn that your emotions are too strong and require that you distance yourself until you can better regulate an emotion. When emotions are overly strong, time to reflect may be the foremost component that is necessary for self-regulation.

The first step in self-regulation is discovering actions that help reset your emotional state. These actions vary somewhat from person to person, so it is important to reflect on your own strategies and work to build a toolbox of self-regulating behaviors and strategies. Here are a few strategies that may work to bring that emotional temperature back to a moderate level: deep breathing, meditation, visualization, walking, getting a drink of water, stretching, exercise or yoga poses. These actions take a few minutes and allow the body and mind to reset. Often, time is the factor that allows for reflection and awareness of the emotional role of the response. This is not an exhaustive list by far. To improve your self-regulation, you should think about strategies that have worked for you in the past and consider some new strategies that allow time for your rational thought to impact your emotional response. Next time you note a change in your emotional temperature that needs a reset, try one of these strategies and see how it works for you.

The second focus of self-regulation is knowing when to stop an action or walk away from a situation that will not have a positive outcome in your current emotional state. Let's face it, sometimes that emotional temperature takes time to reset, or there is a valid reason why your emotional temperature is hot or cold, and you need time to sit in that emotion. That is perfectly understandable. The difference for individuals with high emotional intelligence is that they use their self-awareness and self-regulation to recognize that they need to remove themselves from a situation. They realize that they need to take the time to process the emotion and allow the rational brain to speak. This allows a response to the situation that reflects sound logic and a moderate emotional temperature.

Consider this scenario: You are working in an acute care hospital and are assigned to work with a patient receiving chemotherapy for breast cancer. You recently lost a close friend to breast cancer who was the same age as the patient you are about to see. Just reading their chart brings a wave of emotions and causes you to become very sad and tearful. You take a short walk down the hall and some deep breaths because you know that these strategies help you reset your emotional temperature. After you calm down, you go to the patient's room. But as you go to enter the room, you look at her, and she closely resembles your dear friend, and the feelings return. Using self-regulation, you realize that the patient will not receive the best care from you at this moment because of your emotions. Instead of pushing through it without crying, you contact a coworker, quickly explain the situation, and ask to switch patients. On your walk to the next patient, you reset and are able to provide the next person with great care, and the initial patient also receives great care from your coworker. Using your self-awareness and self-regulation strategies in this scenario provided the best outcome for everyone. You may find that with time and rational thought, you can prepare yourself to work with similar patients in the future without this initial strong emotional response.

Self-motivation – The third component of emotional intelligence is self-motivation. This component builds on your self-awareness and self-regulation to help you stay focused on tasks and outcomes by combining the other two components to move forward. Consider this scenario: You have a big project due for a class at the end of the week, an upcoming exam in a difficult class, and you realize that your best friend is leaving for an internship for the next three months. Your self-awareness and self-regulation allow you to realize that these events have the potential for heightened emotions and potential for derailing your focus. Self-motivation allows you to start planning and give yourself the bandwidth to manage these tasks and emotions responsibly. For example, you might make sure you spend time with your friend and say goodbye early in the week. You might schedule study time while making time for sleep and exercise to keep your body and mind focused. All these things reflect the self-motivation aspects of emotional intelligence and demonstrate effective goal setting that considers emotions and stress response. They are also the foundational building blocks of resilience discussed later in Chapter 6.

By now, you have ways to start building your personal components of emotional intelligence. Once you take the time to work on these areas and strengthen your emotional intelligence foundation, it's time to move from your personal emotional intelligence skill set to the social components of emotional intelligence.

Reflection Moment

Consider the following:

1. In what ways are you in tune with your emotional temperature?
2. Describe a time when you didn't realize the impact of your emotional temperature on a situation.
3. Describe a time when you practiced self-awareness, self-regulation, or self-motivation to handle the emotions of a situation.
4. What activities do you use to self-regulate your emotions?

Set Your Intentions

Think about the questions above and consider how you can integrate some activities into your day to improve your self-awareness and self-regulation of emotions. Now think of your future plans. Do you see an activity that might be influenced by emotions? If so, what strategies will you use to reduce the impact of emotions on that activity?

Social Components

Have you ever met someone who just seems to "get" other people? You know who I mean… the person who seems to have a deep understanding of self and others, someone that others go to for help in gaining perspective on people and situations. This person can often read a room and skillfully manage the emotional temperature. This person has strong emotional intelligence. And whether they actively recognize it or not, they are utilizing practices and skills that reflect the social components of emotional intelligence.

The Role of Empathy – A hallmark of social emotional intelligence skill is the ability to use empathy. Empathy is the ability to place oneself in the emotional place of another. This skill allows health care clinicians to connect more deeply with their patients and team members. It's important to differentiate empathy from sympathy. Empathy is not feeling sorry for someone or relating your similar experience to their current experience. Empathy requires you to place yourself in the feelings of others without judgment and to visualize their experience. It requires awareness and regulation of your feelings as well as the feelings of others. Remember, at the beginning of this chapter, we stated that emotional intelligence is a learned behavior. You, too, can have these same skills by practicing the components. Let's look at each a bit more closely.

Social-awareness – The presence of emotionally intelligent social awareness means that you are able to pick up clues from others that inform you of their current emotions and the temperature of those emotions. What's important here is that we also recognize when our own bias or emotions skew the readings of these emotions. This is why having a strong foundation of self-awareness is important for building social awareness. Consider some examples: Have you ever felt that someone was angry at you or frustrated with you, and when you asked them about it, they weren't angry or frustrated at all? In this scenario, you likely projected your own emotions and/or bias into the situation and misread the scenario. Likewise, if you ever walked into the room and felt the tension between others and quickly saw the signs of this tension, such as someone storming out of the room, you had a good read on the emotions of others.

So how does someone learn social-awareness skills? Social awareness takes some of the same skills as self-awareness but builds on it with strategies such as active listening. Active listening can help us to build our understanding of others, which is the foundation of empathy. You may want to improve your social awareness by simply allowing time to debrief with yourself or a peer after a social interaction such as a patient encounter or team conference. Pause after each interaction with others and consider the potential emotions of others in the room. This is a time where mentoring becomes a helpful tool. If a mentor or a trusted peer is also involved in this encounter, check in with them and compare their assessment of the situation. Did you both read the situation in a similar manner? Did you observe the same emotions? If not, what clues led each of you to your assessment? As an emerging professional, activities such as debriefing interactions with more experienced clinicians can help you grow in your social awareness of emotional responses within individual engagement and team dynamics. Similar to the journaling suggested for personal self-awareness, a helpful tool for building social awareness is to keep a journal of professional interactions and reflect on them to see how interactions can be impacted positively and negatively as you manage the relationship between emotions and rational thought. These reflections help to build your understanding of the complexity of emotional responses in health care. Once you feel more comfortable with identifying the emotional temperature of others around you, it's time to consider social regulation.

Social-regulation – Self-regulation is one of the more complex components of emotional intelligence because it requires combining the skills of regulating your emotional response while also recognizing and understanding the emotional response of others. Just as active listening creates social-awareness, it is an invaluable tool in building social-regulation. This entails listening to truly hear the person, not just to formulate a response, and then asking follow-up questions that allow you to clarify and build the story of their emotions in your mind. Active listening also provides an opportunity to push aside your emotions and biases that may cloud your observation of the person's true emotional temperature. The goal of active listening is to then formulate a response that is reflective and sensitive to the emotional state of another. It allows you to manage a situation with emotionally supportive language that helps create and maintain healthy relationships. Research also supports the role of humor in health care interactions and its role in making challenging situations more comfortable for patients.[5,6] You may know someone who has learned to use respectful humor to reduce tension or uplift others. When using humor, it is important to be aware of context and audience.

Another skill that aids active listening is motivational interviewing. Motivational interviewing is a technique that encompasses active listening and empathy. It is a communication tool, often discussed and utilized in health care, to establish rapport and explore the relationship between values and beliefs and their impact on patient/client behaviors. Motivational interviewing skills suggest that a practitioner utilize open-ended questions, listen actively, affirm the answers, reflect, and then establish a shared understanding. It offers a strategy that allows the patient to truly be understood.[7] For example, consider a patient who is frustrated and sad because they were progressing in their mobility all last week, and this weekend, they tried a bit more activity, and their pain returned. A therapist may use skills such as active listening or motivational interviewing to understand how the patient feels about their setback. In utilizing active listening and motivational interviewing skills, the therapist can understand the patient's frustration and sadness and maybe even state, "I see

how this would be really frustrating," thereby demonstrating an empathic approach to patient interaction.

Consider the skills discussed in Chapter 4 on effective communication and how to use these strategies to enhance your awareness of how others respond. Consider the case study between Payton, George, and Julia and think about how Payton used communication strategies such as non-verbal skills, active listening, and changing their instructions based on George's and Julia's DISC communication styles. As an influencing clinician, Payton regulated the social interaction by having strong self-awareness and regulation of their own tendencies and, in turn, provided communication in a manner that kept everyone's emotional temperature at a moderate level. Reflecting on this case study shows the complexity of skills required for effective social regulation in health care. It demonstrates why it is important to incorporate emotional intelligence learning strategies into professional development.

Empathy, active listening, and motivational interviewing require practice and reflection. They aid in developing skills that build rapport and support that are useful in managing conflict and building concordance. Emerging professionals can build social-regulation skills by journaling and engaging in self-reflection, and finding opportunities to be mentored by reflective and influencing clinicians.[8] Refer to **Figure 5.2** to review the components of emotional intelligence.

Reflection Moment

Consider the following:

1. In what ways are you aware of the emotions of those around you?
2. Have you ever explicitly used active listening? If yes, explain how it impacted your understanding of another. If not, take some time over the next week to actively listen to others.
3. Describe a time when you helped someone bring their emotional temperature to a moderate level.
4. Consider some reflective phrases that show that you "hear" the emotions of another.

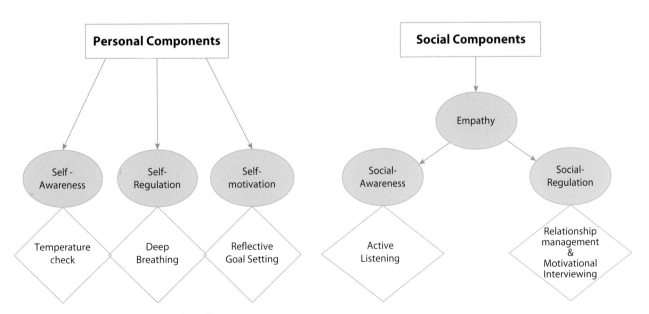

FIGURE 5.2. Components of Emotional Intelligence.

Set Your Intentions

Think about the questions above. What skills did you use or not use in these situations? How might journaling or a mentor help you improve your abilities to understand and guide others' emotions?

● ASSESSING EMOTIONAL INTELLIGENCE

In this chapter, we discussed the components of emotional intelligence and how individuals can work to improve their awareness and regulation in personal and professional situations. To better understand yourself, it may be helpful to measure your current level of emotional intelligence. Several tools exist which examine the components of emotional intelligence. Employers and professional development coaches often use these types of tools in development programs and coaching sessions. Having insight into your emotional intelligence metrics provides a coach or mentor with a foundation on which to develop specific and individualized professional development plans. **Table 5.1** gives a brief overview of a few of the emotional intelligence assessment tools available.

As shown in Table 5.1, the type of tools available to measure emotional intelligence vary including self-reporting, peer input, and ability-based tools. Although all of the tools listed are valid and reliable, caution should be used with self-assessment tools because of the potential for self-reporting bias. Self-assessment tools such as the Emotional Quotient Inventory (EQ-i) and the Schutte Emotional Intelligence Scale (SEIS) help measure change over time and can be used to establish development goals as long as you are aware of your personal bias when completing. The Emotional Confidence Inventory consists of feedback to a third party from supervisors, peers, and subordinates. This type of tool is beneficial for employers and in mentoring and coaching programs. We will discuss 360 evaluation in more detail later in this book. The Mayer-Salovey-Caruso Emotional Intelligence Test (MSCEIT) provides a measure of emotional intelligence that works to eliminate self-bias and feedback from others. This tool is ideal for research projects but may be too involved for individual professional development. Although all assessment tools have limitations, when used as a component of professional development, they serve as a way to gather a more objective measure of emotional intelligence and provide a starting point for goal setting within a professional development plan.

● SUMMARY

This chapter demonstrates how emotions play a significant role in all aspects of our life. From our daily interactions to important decisions, emotions influence our actions, thoughts, and relationships with others. In the health care environment, emotions can have life-altering effects on patients and health care providers. An awareness of the role of emotions in our lives and strategies to incorporate appropriate emotions into our interactions are necessary tools in health care delivery. We have explored the basics of emotions, the definition of emotional intelligence, the components that make up emotional intelligence, and some assessment tools that can be used for emotional intelligence development throughout our professional careers. Now let's apply this knowledge to case studies and personal strategic development.

● CASE STUDIES

As physical therapy professionals, we can set our intentions to apply lifelong learning to the skill of emotional intelligence. Not only will this help us grow in our personal lives, but as the literature points out, emotional intelligence may enhance our careers and improve our interactions with patients, peers, business associates, and the community. In this section, we examine four case studies focusing on the components of emotional intelligence.

CASE STUDY 1
Patient/Client: I can't wait to go on my honeymoon!

Remi is a physical therapist working in an outpatient clinic. They are working their last day before they have two weeks off for their wedding and honeymoon. Remi feels like they are floating through the day. They can't believe their wedding is finally here and that they will soon be on their honeymoon in Hawaii! Remi walks toward the next patient's treatment room with a light skip in their gait.

TABLE 5.1. Emotional Intelligence Assessment Tools[3,4,9]		
Assessment Tool	**Type of Assessment**	**Description**
Emotional Quotient Inventory (EQ-i)	Self-Assessment	133 items on a 5-point Likert scale A shorter version of 52 items Children's version for children ages 7-15
Schutte Emotional Intelligence Scale (SEIS)	Self-Assessment	33 items reported on a 5-point Likert scale
Wong and Law Emotional Intelligence Scale (WLEIS)	Self-Assessment	16 items reported on a 7- point Likert scale
Emotional Competence Inventory	360-Assessment From peers, supervisors, direct reports	Interview style
Mayer-Salovey-Caruso Emotional Intelligence Test (MSCEIT)	Ability-based test Includes tasks such as rating the extent and type of emotion in a picture	Examines: perceiving emotion, facilitating thought, understanding emotions, managing emotions

TABLE 5.2. Case Study 1—Components of Emotional Intelligence

Component	Remi's Approach
Self-awareness	Remi's emotional temperature is high as they are overly happy about the upcoming positive events in their life. This is evident in the nonverbal cues. It is important for Remi to do a temperature check and be aware that this may not be conducive to the emotions of their patient.
Self-regulation	In this situation, once Remi recognizes their emotional temperature, they will need to pause, take a deep breath, and proceed while appearing calmer and less joyful before entering the room.
Self-motivation	In this situation, Remi will need to reflect and realize that the overall goal is to keep the focus on the treatment goals.
Empathy	Remi can use visualization to understand Ali's emotions better and drive the interaction with compassion and understanding.
Social-awareness	In the past sessions, Remi knows that Ali has been very emotional. It is important for Remi to take time and explore Ali's emotional state before starting the therapy session. She can do this by actively listening without judgment.
Social- regulation	Once Remi becomes aware of Ali's emotional state, they may need to use motivational interviewing and continued active listening to recognize and manage Ali's emotional response to the interaction.

Ali is Remi's next patient. She is a 35-year-old woman who has recently been diagnosed with breast cancer. Following surgery, Ali developed lymphedema and cervical pain. It's been a tough few months for Ali. She has missed many things in her life, including a recent family vacation.

Over the past few weeks of treatment. Remi and Ali have really connected. They are the same age and have similar interests. Ali has confided in Remi during her treatments about her frustrations with her medical status and the challenges she has faced in her life. As Remi heads towards the room, they briefly review Ali's chart. They recall that during the last session, Ali had a lot of pain and was very tearful.

In **Table 5.2**, we consider some of the emotional intelligence components of this case study

 EMERGING PROFESSIONAL

As an emerging professional, Remi has gained skills in both self-awareness and self-regulation. They understand the importance of needing to be calm and engaging with patients. In this situation, Remi, takes a few deep breaths and brings down their overly happy mannerisms, such as the skip in their gait. Remi gets mentally prepared that Ali may not be in a good mood and may be tearful. Although Remi has developed self-management skills in emotional intelligence, they find reading all of the cues from patients and helping patients reset their emotions to be challenging in the short time they have with their patients. As Remi starts to engage with Ali, they may find that they cannot redirect Ali's tearfulness and are not able to get Ali through her treatment program. Although Ali still completed components of her treatment session, she may leave the physical therapy clinic still feeling tearful and not feeling that she is making good progress towards her goals.

 REFLECTING PROFESSIONAL

As a reflecting professional, Remi builds upon their self-awareness and self-regulation and checks in with their own emotional temperature throughout the day. Remi has well-developed self-regulating skills and takes time at the beginning and end of each day to reset their emotional

temperature. At the end of the day, Remi writes in a journal and reflects on situations they handled well and ways to improve their interactions. Before starting work each day, Remi reflects on previous encounters with patients they plan to see. Remi had reviewed their journal thoughts on the last session with Ali and recalled that the session required a calm and focused approach. Remi makes a mental note to do some deep breathing and visualizations to capture a very calm emotional state for themselves prior to their time with Ali.

Through collaboration with peers and continuing education, Remi has more confidence in working through challenging conversations with patients and supporting them while still keeping themselves and the patient focused on the goals of a treatment session. Remi's growth in this area helps to reduce the amount of energy they need to help regulate the emotions of patients throughout the day. However, Remi finds that this process still requires preparation and focus. For example, Remi writes down open-ended questions that reflect motivational interviewing skills prior to working with patients so that they recall how to use them and to keep the conversation moving. They find that they must pause and take a deep breath to calm their thoughts before actively listening. With ongoing practice, Remi will continue to develop these motivational interviewing skills and continue to grow in social regulation. Through Remi's preparation, they now have a few open-ended questions that have worked with patients in similar situations in the past. Remi jots down these questions as a resource for Ali's sessions. Remi also considers some potential key goals for Ali's sessions to keep them focused and moving forward. This preparation process helps Remi prepare for emotionally charged sessions.

 INFLUENCING PROFESSIONAL

As an influencing professional, Remi is able to reset their emotional temperature from patient to patient quickly. Knowing that they may need a calm and quiet disposition with one person, use humor and fun with another, and still may need a bit sterner interaction with someone else.

Because Remi has grown in their emotional intelligence, they are able to move through these emotional states seamlessly. Remi also realizes that it is important to stay focused on the goals for each patient's sessions in order to stay focused on outcomes and not allow emotions to derail the interaction. For example, Remi knows that using humor can lead to a lot of fun chatter and discussion and use up too much of the patient's treatment time. So, they carefully use humor as a motivator but not a distraction. In this situation, Remi knows that they must approach Ali with calm emotions and use caring and open body language to engage Ali. Remi also reviewed Ali's chart before entering the room and knows that Ali wanted to work on being able to tolerate short walks with her dog this month. Remi plans to use this goal to keep the session focused on recovery.

Remi is very skillful at understanding others' emotional temperatures. They begin sessions with open-ended questions regarding how the person feels about their progress in therapy and overall health and well-being. They carefully reflect on what the other person is saying to clarify details and understand their perspective. In this way, Remi uses empathy and visualization to truly understand their patients. Once they have a good understanding, Remi has developed their skills in motivational interviewing to discover the individual's strategies for motivation. For example, by using motivational interviewing, Remi may discover that Ali is really frustrated that her family doesn't understand her pain levels and how it impacts her ability to engage in daily life. From this interaction, Remi knows that one of the things they need to add to the session today is ways for Ali to have these discussions with loved ones. After this discussion, Ali's mood improved, and she became open to focusing on physical therapy activities. Remi takes the time to discuss Ali's primary goal with her to ensure they are on the same page. Once they confirm that Ali's goal of walking the dog is important, Remi discusses how current physical therapy activities relate to achieving that goal.

Remi's use of emotional intelligence set the stage for a positive physical therapy session and provided emotional support to Ali. Ali left her physical therapy session feeling positive about reaching her goals with some strategies to use when feeling frustrated in the future.

CASE STUDY 2
Peers: I just can't bear to listen to one more person today!

Monika recently accepted a new position as a clinic director for a skilled nursing facility rehabilitation department. Monika knew she would face challenges in this role. The last director left over six months ago, and since that time the staff has become frustrated with the facility management and each other. Although Monika had opportunities in her education and personal life to lead others, this was her first official leadership role. Monika knew it would take a lot of self-management to be successful and build a strong team culture.

The first few weeks in her new role flew by and Monika felt as though she was getting to know the team and

building connections. She made a few small changes in the department and believed that the changes were well received and the team respected her decision-making process. Monika had gotten into the habit of journaling every few days about her experience to keep her grounded and focused on her goals.

On one particular day, Monika began with a busy morning schedule. She started her day in the facility leadership meeting, where she listened to several complaints regarding her team's interaction with the nursing staff. After that meeting, she knew she needed to think and regroup, so she took a short walk through the facility. Her next responsibility was a meeting with a family who was very upset about the lack of progress their loved one was making. She knew this would require management through a lot of emotions. After making it through the very tearful family meeting, Monika then visited a patient in their room regarding a complaint. She could tell that the patient was very agitated and found all of her emotional energy to help calm the patient and listen to their concerns regarding a negative interaction between a nursing aide and a therapist. After supporting the patient and working to motivate the patient to participate in the next treatment session, Monika decided that she needed to wait until after lunch to address the patient's concerns.

Monika headed back to her office where she had intentionally scheduled an hour to regroup from her roller coaster morning and prepare for the afternoon. Monika expected a busy afternoon and knew she would need to build up her emotional energy to complete her day. Just as she sat down, Shanel, a physical therapist, walked into Monika's office and started to tell her about a recent confrontation with a nurse. Shanel was visibly upset. As she spoke, Monika could feel her own emotional temperature rise. She could tell that she was feeling angry and frustrated with the nursing team and what felt like an ongoing battle between the two departments. Logically, Monika knew that this was not the case and that both teams were experiencing challenges. She also knew that she needed to approach this from a calm emotional state if she was going to be successful in building a team culture within her department and facility. As Monika continued to listen, she knew that her anger was getting the best of her. Monika was at a critical point in her emotional self-management. In **Table 5.3**, we consider some of the emotional intelligence components of this scenario.

 EMERGING PROFESSIONAL

As an emerging professional, Monika gained skills in self-awareness and self-regulation and put a strategy in place to maintain motivation towards her goals. Monika also developed skills for social awareness and social regulation. She knows social skills take a lot of her energy and that she needs to use strategies to regroup her own energy to be present for others. Monika knew that this was a skill she would need to continue to develop in order to successfully lead the team and build a strong culture.

TABLE 5.3.	Case Study 2—Components of Emotional Intelligence
Component	**Monika's Approach**
Self-awareness	Monika's emotional temperature is high. Monika has generally experienced an elevated emotional temperature several times throughout the morning.
Self-regulation	Monika used several techniques throughout the day to help manage her emotions, such as deep breathing, regrouping while walking to the next meeting, and blocking time off in her schedule for reflection and planning.
Self-motivation	Monika started a journal to keep her focused on her goals. This practice allows Monika to keep her vision and goal of building a strong team culture as she faces daily challenges.
Empathy	Monika uses active listening and visualization to understand the perspectives of all interactions within her day.
Social-awareness	Monika applied her social awareness skills throughout the day, allowing her to sense other individuals' elevated emotional temperature and the impact on their interactions. She is acutely aware of Shanel's elevated emotional temperature and will need to decide how best to respond.
Social-regulation	Monika used several strategies throughout her day to facilitate social-emotional regulation. She redirected the frustration of the nursing manager in the team meeting by calmly accepting the team's criticism and promising to investigate and come up with solutions. She comforted tearful family members in the family meeting and finally listened to the patient, promised action, and helped to redirect energy to a positive treatment session. Now Monika must support Shanel in regulating her emotions regarding the recent interaction with the nursing team.

In this scenario, Monika feels both her ability to manage her own emotions and the emotions of others waning. In the interaction with Shanel, Monika has difficulty controlling her emotional temperature and begins to feel angry about the nursing situation. She starts to share the nursing supervisor's comments from the leadership meeting. This makes Monika feel more connected to Shanel but also increases their anger towards the nursing team. In this moment, Monika depleted her ability to self-regulate and, therefore, could not help Shanel work through her anger. Monika reflected on this situation in her journal later that day. She realizes that she has put her goal of building a team culture with nursing back a few steps because she overshared during a time of frustration. Monika knows that she must revisit this situation with Shanel and refocus on the goal of building a team culture.

Monika knows that she is developing her emotional intelligence as a professional but realizes that she needs to make sure she is intentional about her development. This situation demonstrates that Monika has steps she can take to improve both her self- management and her social management. In her journaling exercise, Monika sets goals for gaining mentorship and formal training in emotional intelligence.

 REFLECTING PROFESSIONAL

As a reflecting professional, Monika has well-developed self-management and social management skills. Experience and leadership development courses have given Monika insight into strategies to stay calm during challenging interactions and to use empathy to understand other perspectives. In doing so, Monika quickly realizes the challenges the nursing team is facing and how the rehab team may sometimes add to the challenges through their processes. By having this empathic insight, Monika did not feel

emotionally drained by her conversations in the leadership meeting and the other challenging interactions in her morning. When Shanel came into Monika's office, she had the ability to quickly recognize Shanel's emotional state and help her to calm down and work on problem-solving solutions. Later that day, Monika wrote in her journal and reflected on the times she used empathy to work through a challenging interaction. Monika noted what empathic statements had the most impact on the conversation and made plans to leverage this strategy more often.

Monika is aware of the need to continue to gain emotional intelligence to grow as a professional. Therefore, Monika ensures that she has tangible strategies in place to develop her emotional intelligence. She seeks out mentorship and insight from peers who demonstrate strong emotional intelligence, and she looks for resources such as courses, books, and research that give her insight into improving her emotional intelligence.

INFLUENCING PROFESSIONAL

As an influencing professional, Monika participated in several leadership development courses and worked to gain motivational interviewing strategies for patient and peer interactions. Monika spent time journaling throughout her career and has developed many methods to maintain a calm even temperature in most situations. Monika is known to be the leader others turn to for a rational, calm approach to problems. She knows that directing others with the answer and giving solutions is not the best approach to managing emotionally charged interactions. She uses open-ended questions to explore how others are genuinely perceiving the situation. She takes the time to reflect on what she hears from others, asks continued clarifying questions and works to not place her own bias on the emotions of others. These strategies allow Monika to connect with team members and build strong working relationships. She has found that there is less emotional fluctuation in her workday because of her calm and reflective approach to situations. Monika realizes that these strategies reduce the number of challenging situations in her day-to-day interactions with others.

At this level of professional growth within this scenario, Monika has an insightful conversation with the nursing leadership in the management meeting and finds two key areas where the nursing team and the rehab team can change processes to make everyone's life a bit more efficient. Both the nursing manager and Monika leave the meeting feeling a sense of accomplishment. In the family meeting, Monika applies open-ended questions, active listening and reflection to empathically engage the family members. The family shares their fears of future caregiving and family dynamics with Monika and the other team members. From there, the team moves forward with a solid discharge plan that supports the patient and the family members. Monika continues to use her well-developed social regulating skills to engage with the next patient and manage the patient's complaint. Because Monika has built a collaborative connection to the nursing director, she is able to ask the nursing director to meet with the patient and Monika to find a solution to the issue together.

Finally, when Monika interacts with Shanel, she is energized and easily leverages her skills in motivational interviewing to understand Shanel's perspective on the nursing team interaction. Because she has already worked with nursing to solve some of the process issues, Monika is able to share this positive outcome with Shanel and engage Shanel in future problem-solving and team culture. Shanel leaves the discussion feeling as though she was heard and that there is an active way she can help to make the situation better.

Influencing professionals work to build strong emotional intelligence skills and are aware that they never stop growing and learning in this area. Each day and each interaction continue to be a learning experience. They approach emotional intelligence from a place of humility and work to learn from each interaction. Strategies such as journaling and reflection, asking for peer input on their behaviors, and continual knowledge acquisition continue to guide the influencing professional in their life-long emotional intelligence journey.

CASE STUDY 3
Business Associate: The team is not getting anywhere

Let's revisit the case study from chapter four when Michaline, Yolanda, and Rachelle had a challenging interaction on a video conference call. We explored the interaction from a communication perspective. Now, consider it from an emotional intelligence perspective.

Daryn, the director of an inpatient rehabilitation hospital, recently assigned Michaeline, a physical therapist (PT), Yolanda, an occupational therapist (OT), and Rachelle, a speech-language pathologist (SLP) to work collaboratively on developing a new clinical pathway for patients diagnosed with Parkinson's disease. Michaeline is a recent graduate of a clinical neuroscience fellowship that she completed immediately following graduating from her Doctor of Physical Therapy program. Yolanda has more than ten years of clinical experience, primarily working with children in the school system, but in the past year decided to move into adult rehab, and Rachelle is the lead therapist for the SLP program's neuro team.

The three individuals decide to meet via video conference since each works different hours in different parts of the building. The video conference meeting style allows meeting flexibility without significantly impacting everyone's schedule. The first few meetings get off to a challenging start with some technical issues and interruptions. The team decides to break up some of the research and development of the program to work more efficiently. Each team member shares their findings and suggestions when they return to the next call. Michaeline starts by reviewing several pages of in-depth research regarding the historical overview of clinical pathways and concludes with a suggestion that they conduct a pilot trial of several different methods before moving forward. Yolanda is lost halfway through Michaeline's explanation. She interrupts Michaeline several times during her review to express how she feels about the information and suggests they should pick a pathway and see if everyone on the team thinks it is a good idea. Finally, Rachelle, who believes she should lead the way since she is already a team leader for SLP, has outlined a pathway that she believes will lead to the most efficient and effective method. She thanks Michaeline and Yolanda for their work on the project but, after listening to their input, believes that she will take her pathway to Daryn as the decision from the group. Both Michaeline and Yolanda are extremely frustrated. Michaeline thinks that Rachelle is not expressing respect for research and just wants to do things based on her personal knowledge. Yolanda feels as though Rachelle communicated in a harsh manner and didn't consider either of their feelings. The group ends their conversation briefly as the meeting time on the teleconference runs out. The group ends with no decision and everyone feels frustrated. Two weeks later, when Daryn comes to the group to hear progress, there is no progress to report, and each expresses their frustration with the lack of communication from the others in the group. As the program director, Daryn realizes that although this project has gone off the rails, it is an opportunity for the team to learn from each other and gain valuable insight into how emotional intelligence and skills such as motivational interviewing, active listening, and empathy improve team dynamics.

 EMERGING PROFESSIONAL

It is important to note in this scenario that the three clinicians have a variety of experiences; however, all three had difficulty using emotional intelligence. Experience does not guarantee that emotional intelligence improves. Although experiences enhance emotional intelligence, unless someone actively works to understand and gain skills, emotional intelligence may stagnate.

In the scenario above, none of the participants effectively used self-awareness or self-regulation. Michaeline was focused on getting all of her information out and was not aware that she was overpowering the conversation, Yolanda is acting impulsively and showing frustration regularly, and Rachelle has already decided that her way is the best She is not using any active listening skills to hear what Michaeline or Yolanda are saying. Because the three team members are not actively using self-awareness and self-management emotional intelligence techniques, it is difficult even to attempt to use social management techniques.

As an emerging professional, Daryn has some skills in self-management and social-management. He effectively manages his own emotional response and helps others in a one-on-one situation work through their emotional responses. However, Daryn does not always recognize the need to step into team dynamics to be the calming force in a tough conversation.

Reflection Moment

Questions to consider:

1. How might each team member use self-awareness and self-regulating strategies to better engage with each other?
2. What strategies could you use to establish a clear vision within this group in order to work toward a common goal?
3. How might a reflective leader approach this interaction? Would it have helped to have Daryn involved in the discussion? Why or why not?
4. How might Daryn use motivational interviewing techniques, such as open-ended questions, to facilitate better interaction for the team moving forward?
5. How might each team member build on their self-management skills to facilitate social-management skills?
6. What role did technology play in the team's emotional state?

CASE STUDY 4
Patient/Client: I am so frustrated with my progress

Lee is a physical therapist working for a home health agency. Upon arrival she asks Mr. Chen how he is doing and he replies, "Not so good. I am so frustrated with my health right now. I have been doing everything the doctor told me to do, and I still ended up in the ER last week because I couldn't breathe. I have changed my diet, and I stay away from everything I love to eat and it still doesn't matter!"

Lee notices Mr. Chen's frustration and tries to pick up his spirits by saying, "Oh man, I know that must be tough! But I am sure we can keep working on things and keep you out of the hospital. I bet a bit of exercise will make you feel better and help you to see this in a different light."

Mr. Chen appears even more frustrated and states, "All of you health care people are alike. You just tell me it will be ok, do a few things and walk out the door like everything is going to be OK. I don't even think I want to see any of you anymore. None of it is working."

At this point, Lee knows that the conversation is going in the wrong direction. She needs to use emotional intelligence strategies to turn this discussion around and reset the interaction.

Consider Lee's emotional intelligence in this scenario as a practice exercise. Also, consider the interaction from an emerging, reflecting and influencing professional view.

Complete **Table 5.4** for Lee's current emotional intelligence and how her approach can be directed toward a positive result.

Reflection Moment

Questions to consider:

1. What strategies should Lee use to evaluate her own emotions *p*rior to interacting with Mr. Chen?
2. How might this experience help Lee to grow as a professional?
3. List two or three open-ended questions Lee might use to help Mr. Chen during this difficult time.
4. What additional resources or strategies might Lee seek out following this interaction to help her grow toward becoming an influencing professional?
5. What skills should Lee utilize to manage this interaction as an influencing professional?
6. How might Lee use this interaction to mentor reflective and emerging professionals?

● PERSONAL DEVELOPMENT: EMOTIONAL INTELLIGENCE

Take a moment to reflect on the personal and social components of emotional intelligence and how your emotions play a role in interactions with patients/clients, peers, and the community in which physical therapists interact.

TABLE 5.4. Case Study 4—Emotional Intelligence and Approach

Component	Lee's Emotional Intelligence	Lee's Approach
Self-awareness		
Self-regulation		
Self-motivation		
Empathy		
Social-awareness		
Social-regulation		

Reflection Moment

Consider the following questions:

1. Consider the components of emotional intelligence. Have you previously considered this approach to understanding others?
2. Describe how you currently practice any of these components in interactions with others.
3. How do journaling and reflection improve awareness and growth in emotional intelligence?

After reflecting on these areas, consider your professional development level and complete **Table 5.5**. At what level do you consider yourself? Why?

Planning Moment

Now, let's complete your professional strategic development plan for emotional intelligence in **Table 5.6**. Completing the plan in each chapter helps build your overall professional development strategic plan at the end of the book.

TABLE 5.5. Emotional Intelligence Development

My Current Level of Development

	Emerging	Reflective	Influencing
Self-awareness			
Self-regulation			
Self-motivation			
Empathy			
Social-awareness			
Social-regulation			

TABLE 5.6. Professional Development Plan for Emotional Intelligence

Emotional Intelligence Goals (No More Than 2-3)	Tactics to Accomplish My Emotional Intelligence Goals	The Measure of Success for My Emotional Intelligence Goals	Accountability Partner: Who Will I Share My Goals with, and How Will I Check In with Them?

References

1. Scott J. How healthcare leaders can increase emotional intelligence. *Radiol Manage.* Published online July 2, 2013:11-16.
2. Kihlstrom JF, Cantor N. *Social Intelligence.* Cambridge University Press; 2011:564-581. doi:10.1017/CBO9780511977244.029.
3. Faguy K. Emotional intelligence in health care. *Radiol Technol.* 2012;83(3):237-253.
4. Kim MS, Sohn SK. Emotional intelligence, problem solving ability, self-efficacy, and clinical performance among nursing students: A structural equation model. *Korean J Adult Nurse.* 2019;31(4):380-388. doi:10.7475/kjan.2019.31.4.380.
5. McCreaddie M, Payne S. Humour in health-care interactions: A risk worth taking: Humour in health-care interactions. *Health Expect Int J Public Particip Health Care Health Policy.* 2014;17(3):332-344. doi:10.1111/j.1369-7625.2011.00758.x.
6. Christensen M. Humanizing healthcare through humor: Or how medical clowning came to be. *TDR Drama Rev.* 2020;64(3):52-66. doi:10.1162/dram_a_00942.
7. Miller W, Rollnick S. *Motivational Interviewing: Helping People Change.* 3rd ed. Guilford Press; 2013.
8. Sterrett E. *The Role of Empathy in Emotional Intelligence.* HDR Press Inc; 2014. https://www.hrdpress.com/site/html/includes/items/REEI.html#:~:text=Such%20awareness%20or%20ability%20to,all%20areas%20of%20their%20lives. Accessed August 9, 2022.
9. Brackett MA, Mayer JD. Convergent, discriminant, and incremental validity of competing measures of emotional intelligence. *Pers Soc Psychol Bull.* 2003;29(9):1147-1158. doi:10.1177/0146167203254596.

chapter 6

Resilience and Grit

Health care professionals face many challenging situations. They often face emotionally charged interactions back-to-back without time to re-energize while also dealing with life-related tasks and responsibilities. Chapters 4 and 5 discussed ways to effectively manage communication and emotions during health care interactions. Often, there are more requirements than effective communication and self-management to continue to move forward during times of challenge, hardship, and setbacks. What makes some push on when challenged and others decide to step back? Is this drive something one can develop or something we are born with? If we can develop this ability, how do we manage that? The answer to these questions lies in understanding resilience and grit. The study of resilience and grit points to positive connections among job satisfaction, reduced job stress, persistence in a career, and burnout.[1] In this chapter, we define resilience and grit, explore their role in health care and professional development, and examine ways to assess and develop strategies to support resilience and grit.

DEFINING RESILIENCE AND GRIT

The term resilience relates to the capacity of a system, group, or individual to thrive and maintain a core purpose in the face of adversity.[1,2] In other words, resilience is our ability to bounce back after a struggle or failure. When considering resilience, we can address it individually and as a group dynamic. For example, an individual may be resilient within a group while the organization struggles. In the same sense, a social group, organization, or society may possess resilience, but the individuals within those groups may have varying degrees of resilience. For this chapter, we will focus on the individual level of resilience; however, since health care is an interactive societal activity, it is essential to understand some fundamental dynamics of group resilience. Therefore, we will briefly explore ways to understand and explore group resilience in health care.

To best understand resilience, we need to understand what makes someone resilient. Research has found that there are five components to resilience, and through understanding and focusing on these components, individuals can strengthen their resilience throughout their lifetime.[1,3] **Table 6.1** briefly outlines the five elements of resilience.

One noted feature of these five resilience components is that they strengthen as we age.[1-3] As we move through life, our experiences provide opportunities to discover our purpose fully, test our self-reliance, and face certain difficulties alone. Although age does play a factor in the development of resilience, it is not the only way we grow our strength. Self-reflection and developing strong support networks exemplify how we build a reserve that adds to resilience. Relationships with mentors and coaches help us balance our views of life and maintain our physical and mental health to have the endurance to sustain through challenges.

Reflection Moment

Consider the following:

1. What are the things that bring meaning to your life?
2. How do the things that bring you meaning create your purpose?

TABLE 6.1. Five Components of Resilience

Component	Definition
Purpose	Meaningfulness in life
Perseverance	Ability to keep going
Equanimity	A balanced view of life
Self-reliance	Belief in your capabilities
Existential Aloneness	Understanding that some experiences must be faced alone

Adapted from Meyers et al., Wagnild & Collins[1,3]

3. Describe a time when you faced a challenging task by yourself. How did that make you feel?
4. Do you consider yourself a glass-half-full or half-empty person? How does this impact your ability to keep a balance in your life?

Grit and resilience are sometimes interchanged and most often discussed together. While resilience is defined through our ability to bounce back after a setback, grit is defined as an individual's ability to maintain effort and consistent interest in pursuing goals.[1,4,5] Grit is passion. Grit is future-focused. Gritty individuals keep pursuing goals and use various strategies to achieve long-term goals. Research has examined grit in multiple settings and found that grit is associated with better performance in job roles and life satisfaction.[1,4] One of the most noted studies on grit conducted by American psychologist Angela Duckworth and colleagues, examined both cognitive (intellectual effort) factors and noncognitive (behavioral and interaction) factors that influenced the success of more than 1,000 West Point Academy cadets. Their findings showed that noncognitive traits such as a higher level of grit were strong predictors of the ability to complete the grueling Beast Barracks, the initial six-week training, and graduate from the academy.[4] Studies, such as this West Point cadet research, point to grit's role in goal achievement and performance. Grit can drive physical, mental, and intellectual results!

Reflection Moment

Consider the following:

Think of a challenging goal or a time when someone may have told you that something you wanted wasn't possible.

1. Did you feel you could change or do something differently to achieve that goal?
2. What strategies did you use to stay focused on the goal even when goal attainment seemed out of reach?
3. What did you learn from these strategies that might help you achieve future goals?

On the surface, defining and recognizing resilience and grit may seem easy. However, as you dive deeper, you can recognize the complexity and the essential role played in our personal and professional development. Research examining the role of resilience and grit in goal achievement and job performance often includes another noncognitive component, mindset. Mindset is a guiding outlook or philosophy that can impact your choices and outcomes. It is usually described as a fixed or growth mindset. A growth mindset is required to tap into one's resilience and grit. A growth mindset establishes the degree to which one believes in the ability to learn and improve. A growth mindset, in which you believe change and development are possible, connects with a higher level of grit and goal achievement. Studies find that having stressors and challenges that one perceives within their control throughout life help to develop a growth mindset.[6,7]

Conversely, a fixed mindset can inhibit grit and resilience. A fixed mindset denotes a way of thinking that suggests that intelligence and behaviors are difficult to change. It is a self-limiting belief that "either you have it, or you don't." Individuals who face everyday challenges significantly out of their control or do not face any challenges tend to have more of a fixed mindset.[6,7] For example, someone challenged in school, who regularly receives low grades and cannot develop an improvement plan, may have a more fixed mindset regarding their academic abilities. In contrast, someone who also receives low grades but can reflect and work to improve may demonstrate more of a growth mindset. The struggle to achieve the goal allowed the second person to connect the ability to change and grow to an outcome.[4] This reflects how a growth mindset is cultivated and the impact of grit and resilience when faced with challenges!

The following section will briefly review current literature regarding the role of resilience, grit, and mindset in the professional development of health care professionals, particularly the physical therapy profession.

RESILIENCE IN HEALTH CARE

The rigorous educational requirements and the constant stressors within the health care environment make health care professionals an ideal group to examine the relationships of resilience, grit, and mindset. Studies examining a broad spectrum of health care professionals exist, including those that look at physicians, nurses, pharmacists, dentists, and allied health professionals, such as physical therapists. These studies often aim to explore how to quantify the right blend of cognitive aptitude and noncognitive traits for successful outcomes in the academic study of each discipline, as well as the overall career trajectory of individuals working in health care. It is important to understand that although resilience, grit, and mindset all play a role in the level of success, it is challenging to quantify precisely the extent that each plays and even more difficult to determine a predictive indicator of success.

Medical schools and other health care education programs have long relied on standard admission criteria, such as undergraduate academic performance and standardized test scores like the MCATS or GREs, to determine the best candidates. Educators know that although these standardized measures tell some of the story, something is often missing. Even those excelling in these standardized measures do not consistently achieve academic or career success. Recently, research has begun to explore more of the noncognitive traits like grit and resilience. For example, a study examining a 12-point grit scale of graduating medical students showed that those with a higher grit score completed medical school faster, had higher test scores, and tended to have a higher class rank.[8] Like many other studies, this research examined students already enrolled in medical school. Therefore, they could not predict the abilities of potential students with higher grit scores and lower measures on other standardized entrance assessments. Studies in nursing, pharmacy, and physical therapy all demonstrate similar findings related to grit and resilience.[1,6,9–11] A study comparing the grade point average and grit of physical therapist students found a positive correlation between the two.[11] Likewise, researchers compared grit, resilience, and mindset to the academic success of physical therapy students at different academic institutions. They found a connection between grit and both academic and clinical placement success. However, they could not ascertain the relationship between resilience and a growth mindset with academic success.[6] The connection between these noncognitive traits and the academic success of health care professionals is an exciting and developing area of research. As more studies explore the relationships, educational institutions will gain additional tools to evaluate future candidates and establish ways to support developing growth mindsets and strategies for resilience and grit.

We are beginning to see the impact of resilience and grit in academics, but what do we know about the resilience and grit of practicing health care clinicians? There are limited studies examining this connection to resilience, grit, and mindset with health care clinicians. Studies looking at the rate of burnout among physicians found some connection between the level of burnout and grit.[12,13] The COVID-19 pandemic created an opportunity to discern the relationship of resilience within chronic work-related stress. Initial studies examining front-line health care workers and the stress caused by the pandemic indicated a connection between the level of burnout and resilience. Resilience has been identified as a component in the management of job-related stress.[14,15]

● HEALTH CARE TEAMS

There is a connection between grit, resilience, and mindset and the academic success of health care students. Likewise, the association also exists in the level of burnout health care clinicians experience. But how do these factors connect to the abilities of the interdisciplinary team? The interdisciplinary team is crucial to successful patient outcomes and day-to-day functioning in many health care environments.

Team resilience relates to the ability of a group to withstand and overcome stressors in a manner that allows for continued team performance.[16] A resilient team not only overcomes stressors but also continues to function as a cohesive unit despite the stressors.

Interestingly, individual team member resilience is not the only factor influencing team resilience. In order to have resilient health care teams, other factors come into play. Resilient teams also require team familiarity, transformational leadership, and members with self-efficacy and social support structures.[16] The concept of a resilient team exemplifies professionalism at the individual, interpersonal, and societal/institutional levels, as described in Chapter 1. Resilient teams first need members who possess a level of resilience, but more is required to guarantee a resilient team. Those team members also need strong emotional intelligence and interpersonal development to develop strong connections and knowledge of each other's strengths and weaknesses. Finally, institutions must identify leaders that facilitate positive team dynamics. The transformation toward a more resilient team occurs when these components connect.

● RESILIENCE, GRIT, AND THE CONNECTION TO PROFESSIONALISM

Although not directly stated in the APTA key documents outlining professional concepts, it is easy to see how resilience, grit, and mindset are essential to our professional ethical standards and values. For example, see **Table 6.2** below. Sometimes in a physical therapist's career, one may need to rely on grit or resilience to fulfill all professional obligations. The COVID-19 pandemic is an ideal example of when physical therapists utilized the traits of grit, resilience, and a growth mindset to continue professional practice in uncertain times. Likewise, the core value of professional duty calls on physical therapists to not only serve immediate patient needs but also to serve the profession as a whole and to meet societal needs related to physical therapy. Yet again, a professional may experience internal and external barriers while attempting to meet these obligations. Overcoming these barriers requires resilience, grit, and a growth mindset.

TABLE 6.2. Examples of Connections to the APTA Code of Ethics for the PT and PTA and the Core Values for the PT and PTA		
APTA Code of Ethics/Core Values	**Definition**	**Connection to Resilience, Grit, and Growth Mindset**
Principle No. 5/Excellence	Physical Therapists/Physical Therapist Assistants shall fulfill their legal and professional obligations. Excellence in the provision of physical therapist services occurs when the physical therapist and physical therapist assistant consistently use current knowledge and skills while understanding personal limits, integrate the patient or client perspective, embrace advancement, and challenge mediocrity.	One may experience challenges or setbacks in fulfilling professional obligations, such as completing documentation, attending conferences, or maintaining license-required continuing education. Staying current in treatment techniques and evidence-informed practice is challenging. Resilience, grit, and a growth mindset give us the ability to maintain our professional obligations.
Principle No. 8/Social Responsibility	Physical Therapists/Physical Therapist Assistants shall participate in efforts to meet the health needs of people locally, nationally, or globally. Social responsibility is the promotion of a mutual trust between the profession and the larger public that necessitates responding to societal needs for health and wellness.	It may be easy to forget our professional duty and ethical principles to meet the health needs of our communities. It may take a growth mindset to find motivation, skills and knowledge as a physical therapist to give back to the community. Or, grit and resilience may be required to advocate for a patient's needs when there seem to be barriers to rehabilitation.

Adapted from APTA[17]

TABLE 6.3. Standardized Assessments of Resilience and Grit

Scale	Description
Connor-Davidson Resilience Scale (CD RISC)	10-item assessment with a 4-point Likert scale
Brief Resilience Scale (BRS)	6-item assessment with a 5-point Likert scale
Academic Resilience Scale (ARS)	30-item assessment with a 5-point Likert scale
Dweck Mindset Instrument (DMI)	16-item assessment with a 6-point Likert scale
Original Grit Scale (Grit-O)	12-item assessment with 5-point Likert scale
Short Grit Scale (Grit-S)	8-item assessment with a 5-point Likert scale

Adapted from Meyers et al., Miller-Matero et al., Alahdabetab[1,9,18]

ASSESSING RESILIENCE AND GRIT

In this chapter, we defined and discussed resilience and grit and then connected them to a growth mindset. We also considered each component within the health care environment and the professional practice of physical therapy. Where do you stand in terms of resilience and grit? Standardized measures are helpful to understand your personal foundation in each of these areas. These measures provide insight into your current levels and allow you to establish growth goals and areas in which to focus your efforts. **Table 6.3** provides a brief overview of a few standardized quantitative assessments for resilience and grit.

Although using a standardized assessment tool is a good way to quantify resilience and grit, it is helpful to use reflection to create a deeper understanding. **Table 6.4** expands upon the five components of resilience mentioned earlier in this chapter by utilizing open-ended reflection questions. Through the quantitative evaluation (standardized assessment tools) and the qualitative evaluation (open-ended reflection), one can understand resilience and grit and ways to build upon them for professional development.

CASE STUDIES

Understanding the role of resilience, grit, and mindset from a personal and a group level is important in the health care environment. In this section, we look at two case studies focusing on (1) personal resilience/grit, and (2) team resilience. Following these case studies, use the reflection questions to gain insight into your development.

CASE STUDY 1
Personal Resilience and Grit

Maria has always been passionate about pediatrics. She wanted to work with children for as long as she could remember. After receiving physical therapy after a sports injury in high school, Maria connected her love for working with children to a future career in physical therapy. From that point on, Maria was dedicated to becoming a pediatric physical therapist. As an average student, Maria worked extra hard for her grades. She often spent time reflecting on how she could be more efficient at studying and would ask teachers for ways to improve. Maria finally saw her dream come true after many dedicated years of studying. She passed her national physical therapy examination and got her first job offer for a pediatric outpatient clinic. Maria wanted to strive for more, so she set her sights on gaining the experience and knowledge necessary to take the exam to become a board-certified pediatric clinical specialist. Maria developed a plan for continuing education and studying in preparation for the exam. Finally, she was ready to take this next step in her career.

Maria was shocked when she received the examination results. She just missed the passing score! She didn't understand! She had done everything she always did to be successful in school. In fact, she was sure she had studied more for this exam than any other exam in her career.

TABLE 6.4. Reflection Questions—Resilience

5 Components of Resilience Characteristics	Open-ended Questions for Reflection
Purpose	1. What gives me meaning in my life/profession? 2. What do I do that others value? 3. Do I have a philosophy that guides me?
Perseverance	1. When I experienced a challenge, did I work through it? How? 2. Do I finish what I begin?
Equanimity	1. Do I more often see challenges as problems or opportunities? 2. Do others see me as someone who takes life in stride? 3. How do I handle disappointment?
Self-reliance	1. Can I count on myself in times of challenge? 2. How would others say I respond to challenging situations?
Existential Aloneness	1. What sets me apart from others? 2. Am I willing to go it alone even when something isn't popular with others? 3. What life changes have I faced, and how have they changed or not changed me?

Adapted from Wagnild[3]

And she was practicing as a pediatric therapist every day! The exam results were a real disappointment for Maria.

As an emerging clinician, Maria has faced some challenges and setbacks. Although she has leveraged self-reflection and mentoring, she has always been fairly confident in her abilities and strategies to succeed academically. Let's consider some questions for Maria at this point in her career:

Reflection Moment

Consider the following:

1. How does this situation create an opportunity for Maria to grow her resilience?
2. How will grit play a role in Maria's next steps?
3. How can Maria leverage a growth mindset to move forward?
4. Now let's consider Maria in the stages of a reflective or influencing clinician; how might her response to this scenario differ?

CASE STUDY 2
Team Resilience

Mark, Bev, Sandra, and Josiah work together in a small rural community hospital. They are the only physical therapy team in a 75-mile region of their small town. The physical therapy department serves the inpatient community hospital patients and the small skilled nursing home next to the hospital. They also provide outpatient services to the community. The team has worked together for years, covering shifts for each other for vacations and other family obligations. They attend parties at each other's homes and spend time together at local community activities outside work. The physical therapy department truly works as a well-oiled machine. Others have commented that the physical therapy team can finish each other's sentences. The physical therapy department director, Sandra, often says she isn't a director because everyone works together so well. The team is very comfortable in their routine and is often on autopilot. Shortly before the COVID pandemic, Jacelyn, a new graduate, moved to the area and joined the team. Jacelyn struggled at first to fit into the rhythm of the department and to feel like a team member. It wasn't that the others wanted to exclude her; they were just so in tune with each other that it took a conscious effort to bring Jacelyn into the group. Finally, after about a year on the team, Jacelyn felt like she belonged. She was getting to know the other members and was included in the out-of-work activities. She was looking forward to growing her connections; however, things were about to become very challenging for the team.

During the COVID-19 pandemic, the small town faced many challenges, and the physical therapy team was no exception. The usual in-sync group found themselves with differing opinions on the approach to working in such an unstable environment and had difficulty delegating the new responsibilities, especially within the most critical areas of patient care in the skilled nursing facility and the hospital's ICU. As the team's newest member, Jacelyn struggled with how to move forward and have her ideas and concerns recognized by the group.

To make it through this challenging time, the physical therapy team needed to rely on their team resilience and personal grit, and bring a growth mindset to each problem they faced. Below are some key discussion points to consider regarding this scenario. Reflect on them personally as if you were Jacelyn in this scenario. Additionally, it may be helpful to discuss and role-play through these questions with classmates or team members.

Reflection Moment

Consider the five components of resilience and the open-ended questions listed in Table 6.4:

1. Reflect on how Jacelyn might consider these when considering her professional duty as a physical therapist.
2. Reflect on how the team as a functioning unit may answer the open-ended questions.

Consider the concepts of team resilience and traits such as familiarity, transformational leadership, self-efficacy, and social support:

1. What areas might challenge Jacelyn as a new team member and emerging professional?
2. In what areas might the team have strengths or weaknesses?
3. Describe what the team needs to leverage to ensure resilience through this challenge.

● PERSONAL DEVELOPMENT: RESILIENCE, GRIT, AND MINDSET

Take a moment to reflect on each of the three areas; resilience, grit, and mindset. Use the activities below to consider if your development level reflects an emerging, reflective, or influencing professional.

Reflection Moment

Resilience: Use Table 6.4 to reflect on the five components of resilience. Take time to write your answers to the open-ended questions.

Grit: Consider a personal goal. How do you stay focused on that goal? Have you been distracted from it? If so, why? What is your plan moving forward to maintain focus on your goal?

Mindset: Write a letter to your future self: In this letter, consider your future identity, and think about the challenges that may arise to achieve that future identity. Describe a plan to work through these challenges and close the gap between your current level and your future self.

Now, let's complete your professional strategic development plan for resilience, grit, and mindset by completing **Table 6.5**. Remember, completing the plan in each chapter helps build your overall professional development strategic plan at the end of the book.

TABLE 6.5. Professional Development Plan—Resilience, Grit, and Mindset			
Resilience, Grit, & Mindset Goals (No More Than 2-3)	Tactics to Accomplish My Resilience, Grit & Mindset Goals	The Measures of Success for My Resilience, Grit & Mindset Goals	Accountability Partner: Who Will I Share My Goals with? How Will I Check In with Them?

References

1. Meyer, G., Shatto, B., Kuljeerung, O., Nuccio, L., Bergen, A., & Wilson, C. R. (2020). Exploring the relationship between resilience and grit among nursing students: A correlational research study. *Nurse Education Today*, 84, 104246. https://doi.org/10.1016/j.nedt.2019.104246.

2. Zolli A, Healy AM. *Resilience: Why Things Bounce Back*. Simon & Schuster Paperbacks; 2021.

3. Wagnild GM, Collins JA. Assessing resilience. *J Psychosoc Nurs Ment Health Serv*. 2009;47(12):28-33. doi:10.3928/02793695-20091103-01.

4. Duckworth A. *Grit: The Power of Passion and Perseverance*. Scribner; 2016.

5. Duckworth AL, Quinn PD. Development and validation of the short grit scale (Grit-S). *J Pers Assess*. 2009;91(2):166-174.

6. Calo M, Judd B, Chipchase L, Blackstock F, Peiris CL. Grit, resilience, mindset, and academic success in physical therapist students: A cross-sectional, multicenter study. *Phys Ther*. 2022;102(6):pzac038. doi:10.1093/ptj/pzac038.

7. Wolcott MD, McLaughlin JE, Hann A, et al. A review to characterise and map the growth mindset theory in health professions education. *Med Educ*. 2021;55(4):430-440.

8. Miller-Matero L, Martinez S, MacLean L, Yaremchuk K, Ko A. Grit: A predictor of medical student performance. *Educ Health Change Learn Pract*. 2018;31(2):109-113.

9. Calo M, Peiris CL, Chipchase L, Blackstock F, Judd B. Grit, resilience and mindset in health students. *Clin Teach*. 2019;16:317-323. doi:10.1111/tct.13056.

10. Richardson S, Scotto M, Belcina MA, Patel R, Wiener K. Grit and academic performance in Doctor of Physical Therapy students. *Internet J Allied Health Sci Pract*. 2020;18(4):1-4.

11. Pate AN, Payakachat N, Harrell TK, Pate KA, Caldwell DJ, Franks AM. Measurement of grit and correlation to student pharmacist academic performance. *Am J Pharm Educ*. 2017;81(6):1-8. doi:10.5688/ajpe816105.

12. Betchen S, Sarode A, Pories S, Stein SL. Grit in surgeons. *World J Surg*. 2021;45(10):3033-3040. doi:10.1007/s00268-021-06222-0.

13. Halliday L, Walker A, Vig S, Hines J, Brecknell J. Grit and burnout in UK doctors: A cross-sectional study across specialties and stages of training. *Postgrad Med J*. 2017;93(1101):389-394. doi:10.1136/postgradmedj-2015-133919.

14. Phillips K, Knowlton M, Riseden J. Emergency department nursing burnout and resilience. *Adv Emerg Nurs J*. 2022;44(1):54. doi:10.1097/TME.0000000000000391.

15. Pooja V, Khan A, Patil J, Chaudhari B, Chaudhury S, Saldanha D. Burnout and resilience in doctors in clinical and preclinical departments in a tertiary care teaching and dedicated COVID-19 hospital. *Ind Psychiatry J*. 2021;30(3):69.

16. Hendrikx IEM, Vermeulen SCG, Wientjens VLW, Mannak RS. Is team resilience more than the sum of its parts? A quantitative study on emergency healthcare teams during the COVID-19 pandemic. *Int J Environ Res Public Health*. 2022;19(12). doi:10.3390/ijerph19126968.

17. Swisher LL, Hiller P, for the APTA task force to revise the core ethics documents. The revised APTA code of ethics for the physical therapist and standards of ethical conduct for the physical therapist assistant: Theory, purpose, process, and significance. *Phys Ther*. 2010;90(5):803-824. doi:10.2522/ptj.20090373.

18. Alahdab F, Halvorsen AJ, Mandrekar JN, et al. How do we assess resilience and grit among internal medicine residents at the Mayo Clinic? A longitudinal validity study including correlations with medical knowledge, professionalism and clinical performance. *BMJ Open*. 2020;10(12). doi:10.1136/bmjopen-2020-040699.

chapter 7

Accountability

Recall a time when your actions didn't meet expectations. Maybe you missed an assignment deadline or forgot to respond to an email. When we make mistakes, we may instinctively want to discover why the error happened. Or, in other words, we may make excuses or blame a situation or someone else for the mistake. In these moments, we use valuable time and resources to validate previous actions instead of dealing with the current reality of the error. Unfortunately, when we spend time blaming and excusing, we are not acting in an accountable manner. This chapter discusses the concept of accountability, how accountability impacts our health care system, and how accountable language and thought can create actionable outcomes.

● DEFINING ACCOUNTABILITY

According to the Merriam-Webster dictionary, "accountability is an obligation or willingness to accept responsibility or to account for one's actions".[1] In theory, accountability seems easy and something we do every day. However, we may not always act in an accountable way and not even realize we are doing it. Furthermore, we might find ourselves wanting to project accountability onto others. Therefore, awareness of what it means to be accountable, recognizing how to use language that promotes accountability, and modeling these behaviors for those surrounding us is essential for professionals, especially health care professionals.

Let's explore what it means to use accountable language. Accountable language begins when we state our current situation without following the statement with reasons, excuses, or emotions. For example, let's go back to that missed assignment. An accountable view of the current reality is, "I missed submitting the assignment," versus an excuse statement such as, "I missed submitting the assignment because my internet went out and I couldn't connect to upload the assignment." In the first statement, stating the current reality without anything attached sets the individual up for action and moving forward. In the second

statement, the person spends time explaining reasons and gets stuck in the past. This thought cycle is counterproductive to moving forward with corrective action. Look at that current reality statement, "I missed submitting the assignment." What would be a forward-thinking solution? Perhaps to reach out to the professor to see if a late submission is possible and then calculating the missed grade to determine options to make up points. Maybe, create a plan that will avoid missing future assignment due dates. The person who uses an excuse statement is stuck in telling the story about why something happened and not finding actionable solutions. A helpful way to consider accountability is thinking about responsibility through a visual demonstration of the rungs on a ladder.

The accountability ladder, as viewed in **Figure 7.1**, helps you think about accountability in different situations, personally and professionally. Consider the three rungs at the bottom of

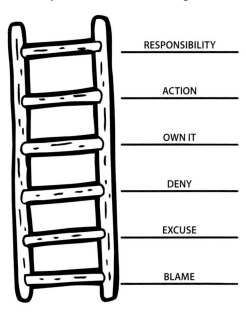

FIGURE 7.1. Accountability Ladder.

the ladder. When using language or a mindset that blames, excuses, or denies a problem, the person is stuck and unable to move upward. However, as soon as the person owns the current reality, they are ready to take action and move toward a position of responsibility. The more one uses this approach, the more they demonstrate active participation and responsibility.

The accountability ladder is a visual demonstration of the concept of internal and external locus of control. An individual who sees the world through an external locus of control believes that things happen to them and around them which are out of their control. Seeing a situation through an external locus of control provides the foundation to place blame, use external reasons or excuses for why something happened, or even deny one's involvement in any part of the situation. Using this approach keeps you stuck at the bottom of the ladder, unable to reach the top rung and move forward. In contrast, an individual who sees the world through an internal locus of control believes that they play an active role in creating the outcomes of situations. These individuals own the current reality and believe their actions impact what happens next. Let's look at an example: A physical therapist is running behind in their clinical schedule. The therapist with an external locus of control view of the world might believe that they are running behind because their patients spent too much time explaining their symptoms, that the office team booked patients who required too much time too closely together, or that they actually weren't behind because the clinical schedule was so unrealistic in the first place. In this example, the therapist is blaming, making excuses, and denying. Also, with this mindset, they cannot change their current reality because the events are external to their control.

Let's look at this example from the internal locus of control. A therapist with an internal locus of control might consider ways to make more time in the schedule. This may require more preparation before seeing the patients each day. It may require rearranging the schedule accordingly to accommodate patient needs and timeframes. Ownership of the situation allows the practitioner with the internal locus of control to move forward, improve the situation, and create positive outcomes.

Everyone has moments when they find themselves stuck on one of the bottom three rungs of seeing the world through an external locus of control lens. In these situations, it's good to reflect on the situation and perhaps even write down the current reality. This mental process helps one to move from inaction to action. So, let's take a moment to reflect on some statements and consider how these statements can be rephrased to create momentum to support moving up the accountability ladder to a level of actionable responsibility.

Reflection Moment

Consider the following health care working examples:

1. Determine what rung of the ladder they currently represent.
2. Restate them as a statement of ownership of the current reality.
3. Determine what might be the following action taken by someone after they own the current reality.

The nurse never called me back to say that Mr. Smith was back from his CT scan, so I didn't see him for his physical therapy appointment this morning.

When they reviewed the vacation request timeline at the staff meeting, I was off sick and missed the deadline for submitting the summer vacation.

There wasn't a blood pressure cuff in the treatment room, so I couldn't take Tom's blood pressure during the evaluation.

I didn't know there was a policy that every patient should have vital signs completed before their treatment session.

Now that you have practiced recognizing when statements blame, excuse, or deny, take some time to reflect on your accountability language. Choose a day in your week to listen to your words and reflect on the following questions.

1. Are there times when you use blame, excuse, or deny statements? If so, what happens in that situation? How do you feel in that situation?
2. Are there times when you recognize your mistake and own your current reality? What are your follow-up actions? How does owning the error and using action to correct it make you feel about the situation?

We should strive for accountable actions in our personal and professional life. Unfortunately, there are times when we don't display accountable actions, and it's essential to have a way to recognize these moments and a strategy to get back to accountability. Although this is important in all aspects of our lives, accountability becomes even more critical when it comes to being a professional in the health care industry. The following section addresses accountability expectations in health care and how owning mistakes and taking corrective actions can improve patient care.

● ACCOUNTABILITY: WHY IT MATTERS IN HEALTH CARE

Mistakes happen in all workplace situations. Health care is no exception. However, errors in the health care profession can produce severe consequences for patients, health care organizations, and team members. It is often confusing and complex when a mistake occurs in patient care. Specific policies and procedures must be followed to communicate mistakes effectively. Most large health care institutions seek legal guidance for significant patient care errors. In environments with such a complex way of dealing with mistakes, the temptation exists to shy away from stating the current reality and to rely on blame, excuse-making, and denial of any adverse action. However, accountability in the health care environment is essential in preventing and correcting errors. It is estimated that medical errors account for nearly 100,000 deaths yearly in the United States and cost approximately $20 billion annually.[2] Medical errors occur in all practice settings, with slightly more than half occurring in outpatient settings.[2]

Consider the accountability ladder discussed in the previous section. Think about what might happen if someone in health care decided to blame someone else for a mistake or deny the issue happened. Not only might this delay a resolution, but consequences may occur for other professionals and the patient when blame or excuses distract from the correct resolution of the issue. Understanding how best to acknowledge mistakes and communicate the next steps in health care is an area explored by researchers and health care legal experts. Many states now have apology laws that help protect health care providers when they openly admit a mistake and say, "I am sorry."[3,4] The research clearly documents that clinicians who apologize for mistakes are less likely to face legal action and have an easier time resolving lawsuits.[3] The fact that laws are necessary to outline the role of an apology in health care demonstrates the complexity of dealing with accountability in the health care environment. Health care professionals need to have resources to help understand the expectations of accountability. For example, professionals in physical therapy can again look to the Core Values of the Physical Therapist and Physical Therapist Assistant, the Code of Ethics for the Physical Therapist, and Standards of Ethical Conduct for Physical Therapist Assistants to define and guide accountability. **Table 7.1** outlines accountability from these guiding documents.

The three documents from the APTA provide a working definition of accountability for the profession and outline the legal, ethical, and sound business obligations of those in the field of physical therapy. For example, physical therapist professionals must self-regulate their actions to ensure positive patient outcomes. Blaming others, using excuses, and denying an issue exists do not allow for self-regulation because the power to act moves externally to the person. Only when we own the current reality of a situation can we move forward with regulating our actions and obtaining a responsible outcome.

● SUMMARY

This chapter defined accountability and the use of the accountability ladder as a guide to understanding the use of accountable language and moving toward actionable outcomes. Using this model as a foundation for decision-making in health care scenarios helps health care professionals understand how to leverage their internal locus of control to recognize problems and mistakes and take positive steps forward to self-regulate their

TABLE 7.1. Accountability from APTA Guiding Documents	
Core Values for the Physical Therapist and Physical Therapist's Assistant	Accountability is active acceptance of the responsibility for the diverse roles, obligations, and actions of physical therapists, including self-regulation and other behaviors that positively influence patient/client outcomes, the profession, and the health needs of society.
Code of Ethics for the Physical Therapist	Principle No. 3: Physical therapists shall be accountable for making sound professional judgments.
Standards of Ethical Conduct for the Physical Therapist Assistant	Standard No. 5: Physical therapist assistants shall fulfill their legal and ethical obligation. Standard No. 7: Physical therapist assistants shall support organizational behaviors and business practices that benefit patients and clients, and society.

Adapted from APTA[5–7]

professional practice. Next, let's apply the accountability ladder to case studies and professional strategic development.

● CASE STUDIES

The more we practice using accountable language and consider which rung of the accountability ladder our words and actions represent, the easier it is to approach daily challenges through an internal locus of control. This section outlines two case studies demonstrating how accountability impacts daily activities in health care. Let's consider both case studies from the perspective of an emerging, reflecting, and influencing professional.

CASE STUDY 1
I am sorry

Beth works in the home health setting and enjoys autonomy and one-on-one time with patients. However, lately, Beth believes that the patients she works with are more fragile and getting less time in the acute care setting before being discharged to home. Beth recently evaluated Mr. Clark following a total knee replacement. Beth was excited to see Mr. Clark's diagnosis on the referral form. Beth thought, "Finally, a straightforward orthopedic patient on my caseload! I never get to see these patients in home health anymore!" During the first treatment session, Beth began Mr. Clark's evaluation, which was like going into auto drive… she didn't have to think and worry about all of the medical complications and frailty that concerned her with her other recent patients. Upon leaving his home, Beth realized that she hadn't done a post-exercise vital sign assessment with Mr. Clark after he ambulated and completed his program. While sitting in her car, she contemplated returning to the home to do a final check and make sure she hadn't missed anything. But then she looked at her watch and realized she had just enough time to run by the office and pick up supplies. She thought, "He looked fine when I left, and I am seeing him in a few days." Beth opted not to collect Mr. Clark's post-exercise vitals and to get on with her day. Before Beth's next scheduled visit with Mr. Clark, she received notice from the office that Mr. Clark had been admitted back into the hospital following a stroke that occurred on the evening of her evaluation. Instantly, Beth had a bad feeling. She had been so excited to work with a patient with a straightforward orthopedic diagnosis that she left her usual caution slip. Not only had she neglected to check Mr. Clark's vital signs after he exercised, she hadn't opened her laptop during the evaluation visit because the battery was low. Beth sat down and looked at Mr. Clark's hospital records again, and there it was… Mr. Clark had a history of hypertension, smoked for over 40 years, and had hypercholesterolemia. The physical therapy notes from the acute care stay stated that exercise was discontinued on two different sessions because of complaints of headaches and elevated blood pressure with activity. Unfortunately, Beth hadn't read any of this information, and Mr. Clark didn't share his medical history because he assumed that his therapist would have access to his records. Beth knew she made a mistake. Although there might not be a direct connection between Mr. Clark's stroke and her evaluation, she hadn't used good judgment. She knew she could easily ignore this information, complete a transfer note, and not say a word about what she missed in the medical record and during her evaluation. She knew she could deny any wrongdoing, and the chances of linking her actions to the outcome were slim. Beth spent the day thinking through scenarios in her head and considered accountability. Let's consider Beth's actions.

 EMERGING PROFESSIONAL

As an emerging professional, this might be the first time Beth has made a significant error when working with a patient. Beth may be tempted to look for external reasons why she did not read the referral documentation or take that last set of vital signs. This may lead to excuses or denial that there was anything she could have done differently. Although these are all possibilities, Beth had a solid education in the Core Values and Code of Ethics and was aware that these documents could guide her to the next steps toward owning the current reality of the situation. Beth may choose to meet with a supervisor or a trusted peer for guidance on the next steps. As an emerging clinician, this process is unnerving, and there are many things Beth has uncertainty about.

 REFLECTING PROFESSIONAL

As a reflecting clinician, Beth builds on the ongoing quality and compliance education she has attended as a working professional. She has worked with patients who experienced medical care errors and witnessed the challenges they face when medical professionals deny wrongdoing. Beth knows that denying her mistake could worsen things for everyone in the long run. She knows she needs to reach out to her compliance officer and supervisor to discuss how to communicate and clearly document her actions with Mr. Clark. Beth is determined to be accountable, follow appropriate policies and processes, and learn from this error in judgment to ensure that this does not happen again.

 INFLUENCING PROFESSIONAL

As an influencing clinician, Beth uses experience and ongoing education to guide her decision-making. Although professionals at all levels of development have bad experiences where they may make errors in judgment, continued education in ethics and an active focus on professional development help Beth in this situation. Although she made an initial error in judgment regarding her relaxed approach to Mr. Clark's care, on her ride back to the office, she considers the possibility that Mr. Clark has other medical concerns. When Beth gets to the office to pick up her supplies, she reviews Mr. Clark's medical records. With awareness of his medical and acute care history, she calls Mr. Clark to check on him and apologizes for omitting post-exercise vitals. She finds that he has access to an automatic blood pressure cuff which she instructs him to use. She carefully reviews exercise precautions and how to seek medical

attention, including a review of emergency numbers. During the discussion, Mr. Clark's blood pressure was in normal ranges, and he was asymptomatic. Beth documents her discussion with Mr. Clark and calls her supervisor to ensure she didn't miss anything else.

CASE STUDY 2
The plan of care wasn't clear

Tavona and Jason have worked together in a skilled nursing facility rehab department for more than a year and have a good working relationship. Tavona is a physical therapist, and in her role, she oversees physical therapy for patients in two different skilled nursing facilities. Jason is a physical therapist assistant responsible for providing physical therapy services at one of the facilities Tavona oversees. Because of her schedule, Tavona is usually only in the facility with Jason for two or three days each week. On the days Tavona is in the building, they meet to review new patients and discuss the plan. However, she always makes sure she is available via phone for any questions per the state practice act guidelines. On the days that Tavona isn't at the facility, they usually check in with each other first thing in the morning and at the end of the day. This past month has been hectic in both facilities, and Tavona has found it challenging to keep up. Jason also felt like the schedule was more demanding. On a few occasions, when Jason called her with a question, it took longer than usual to get back to him, and they had to skip several meetings with each other. This week there were several new patients whom Tavona recently evaluated and Jason planned to see. They hadn't discussed the patients, but Tavona had written her care plan with the flexibility Jason and Tavona expected. She respected Jason's strong clinical judgment and this flexibility allowed for the advancement of exercise and mobility, based on what Jason observed.

Ms. Jones was one of the new patients who started her physical therapy this week. She has a complex medical history and recently had several falls. One of those falls was associated with two rib and thoracic vertebrae fractures. She did not initially complain of pain and wasn't experiencing any shortness of breath or challenges with upper extremity movement. Tavona's care plan was to progress with upper extremity exercise and trunk mobility as tolerated. On her third physical therapy session, Jason added 2-pound weights to Ms. Jones's upper extremity exercises and initiated gentle trunk rotations, side bending, and deep breathing exercises. Ms. Jones tolerated the activity well and had no complaints of pain. Later that day, the nurse called the rehab department, and Tavona, who had just arrived, answered the phone. The nurse informed Tavona that they were ordering X-rays for Ms. Jones because they thought she had a new fracture related to complaints of pain following her physical therapy session.

Tavona was very concerned and questioned Jason about Ms. Jones' program. She thought Jason moved too quickly by adding weights and trunk mobility on the same day and asked why Jason didn't clarify the progression with her. Jason was frustrated with Tavona and stated that if she wanted her to move at such a slow pace, then her care plan should reflect exactly what she wanted Ms. Jones to do, and she should have made a point to talk to him about her care.

In the scenario above, Tavona and Jason view the situation through an external locus of control. They are stuck on the bottom rungs of the accountability ladder. In the following reflections, consider what each of them needs to do to move to owning reality and finding their next action steps. Consider how emerging, reflecting, and influencing clinicians may handle this situation and what skills they would leverage.

Reflection Moment

Consider the actions and language of both Tavona and Jason in this scenario:

1. How can each change their view of this situation from an external to an internal locus of control?

2. Design statements that reflect owning the current reality and moving forward with action.

3. In **Table 7.2**, outline how Tavona and Jason may act as emerging, reflective, and influencing professionals.

The cases presented in this section provide you with a foundation to consider other health care examples of accountability. It is helpful to spend time discussing accountable actions with peers and mentors as well to develop a framework for thinking through accountable actions in your daily professional life. Consider these case studies and other discussions when completing your professional development plan.

● PROFESSIONAL DEVELOPMENT

Now, let's complete your professional strategic development plan for accountability by using **Table 7.3**. You may see how accountability is closely tied to communication with others, emotional quotient, resilience, grit, and mindset as discussed in previous chapters. Remember, completing the plan in each chapter helps build your overall professional development strategic plan at the end of the book.

TABLE 7.2. Case Study 2 Accountable Actions

	Tavona	Jason
Emerging		
Reflecting		
Influencing		

TABLE 7.3. Professional Development Plan for Accountability

Accountability Goals (No More Than 2-3)	Tactics to Accomplish My Accountability Goals	The Measures of Success for My Accountability Goals	Accountability Partner: Who Will I Share My Goals with, and How Will I Check In with Them

References

1. Accountability. https://www.merriam-webster.com/dictionary/accountability.

2. Rodziewics T, Housman B, Hipskind J. *Medical Error Reduction and Prevention*. StatPearls Publishing; 2022. https://pubmed.ncbi.nlm.nih.gov/29763131/#:~:text=Medical%20errors%20cost%20approximately%20%2420,100%2C000%20people%20dying%20each%20year.

3. Lee MJ. On patient safety: do you say "I'm sorry" to patients? *Clin Orthop Relat Res*. 2016;474(11):2359-2361. doi:10.1007/s11999-016-5025-7.

4. Baum NH, Dowling RA. How an apology may help you avoid litigation: Knowing when and how to say "I'm sorry" is vital to patient and physician well-being. *Urol Times*. 2008;36(5):30.

5. Swisher LL, Hiller P, for the APTA Task Force to revise the core ethics documents. The revised APTA code of ethics for the physical therapist and standards of ethical conduct for the physical therapist assistant: Theory, purpose, process, and significance. *Phys Ther*. 2010;90(5):803-824. doi:10.2522/ptj.20090373.

6. Core values for physical therapist and physical therapist assistant HOD P09-21-21-09. Published online December 14, 2021. https://www.apta.org/apta-and-you/leadership-and-governance/policies/core-values-for-the-physical-therapist-and-physical-therapist-assistant. Accessed April 10, 2022.

7. Standards of ethical conduct for the physical therapist assistant HOD Soc-20-31-26. Published online 8/12/2020. https://www.apta.org/apta-and-you/leadership-and-governance/policies/standards-of-ethical-conduct-for-the-physical-therapist-assistant. Accessed February 5, 2023.

chapter 8

Cultural Quotient: Cultural Competence and Cultural Intelligence

The lived experiences of patients and clients vary greatly. Individuals' race, ethnicity, religion, gender, sexual orientation, educational level, disability, and socioeconomic status are examples of ways our diverse identities influence our beliefs, values, norms, and behaviors. These factors impact our interactions, experiences, and outcomes in all aspects of life, including health. Therefore, it is essential for health care providers to gain the perspective of the patient's lived experiences to translate professional knowledge into interaction skills that create positive outcomes. In previous chapters, we discussed understanding the diversity of communication styles, the role of emotional intelligence, and the ability to leverage a growth mindset as a clinician. These skills all work together to assist physical therapy professionals in developing their cultural quotient. In this chapter, we explore the definition and components of cultural competence and cultural intelligence, examine cultural quotient's role in health care, and discuss ways to assess cultural competence and cultural intelligence.

Acquiring skills in understanding and applying culturally appropriate approaches to health care requires clinicians to utilize a growth mindset (Chapter 6), communication strategies (Chapter 4), and emotional intelligence (Chapter 5) to leverage active listening skills and empathy in understanding each person's unique lived experience. Professional development in this area starts with a foundational knowledge of key terms and an awareness of how the concepts build upon each other. Cultural competence and cultural intelligence provide frameworks for thinking about cultural learning.

● DEFINING CULTURAL COMPETENCE

Cultural competence is a set of uniform attitudes, behaviors, and principles that guide the ability to work effectively with people from different cultures. Cultural competence generally consists of five key elements of consideration: ***desire, awareness, knowledge, skill, and encounters***.[1,2] It's important to note that, like professionalism, cultural competence is a lifelong journey. As we encounter more diverse individuals in our lives and the world evolves, the journey through the process continues.

Cultural Desire

The desire to gain cultural competence is this journey's foundational element. Caring is core to the aspiration toward cultural competence. As health care providers, physical therapy professionals care about their patient's well-being. Understanding how others experience the world helps clinicians evaluate and examine, determine a diagnosis, and create a collaborative plan for individualized care. Therefore, physical therapy professionals must maintain a desire to understand patients' perspectives and experiences throughout their careers to ensure individualized care.

Cultural Awareness

"First, know thyself." This ancient Greek advice is core to the next element of cultural competence. Understanding our perceptions and who we are is the first step in gaining cultural awareness. Exploring our own culture and the bias, stereotypes, prejudices, and assumptions our culture has instilled in the lens through which we see the world is critical to gaining cultural awareness. Without this awareness, health care clinicians may use cultural imposition, imposing their beliefs, values, and perspectives into patient engagement. You may have experienced this in your own life. For example, if someone assumed you practiced the same religion or expressed the same political views, or even liked the same sports team as they did without exploring your actual perspective, you have experienced cultural imposition. When we know the origins of our views and understanding of the world, we are less likely to assume others share those views.

Cultural awareness progresses through several levels, beginning with unconscious incompetence. At this level, one is not aware of their lack of cultural knowledge. In essence, they are in a state of blissful ignorance. In this state, they are unaware of cultural differences and do not realize any cultural mistakes. Cultural awareness then moves through three additional levels to the highest level of unconscious competence, in which the individual has gained extensive cultural knowledge and skill and no longer needs to think about interacting in a culturally appropriate manner. This reflects the movement of a professional through the emerging, reflective, and influencing phases of development. Therefore, it is essential to reflect on your level of cultural awareness. **Table 8.1** outlines the four levels of cultural awareness.

Cultural Knowledge

The foundational desire to provide individualized patient care and the awareness of our unique lived experiences, shaped by our culture, gives us the stepping-off point to gain cultural knowledge. This lifelong process entails the acquisition of critical artifacts such as health-related beliefs, cultural practices, and cultural values. Gaining cultural understanding is a goal that physical therapy professionals should incorporate into a personal development plan throughout their careers. The continued acquisition of cultural knowledge aids in developing relationships, gaining trust, and utilizing skills that optimize the provision of appropriate individualized patient care.

Cultural Skill

The ability to empathize and effectively interact with others with cultural awareness and knowledge will be displayed as a cultural skill. Cultural skill is often reflected in our communication and often becomes evident during an initial patient encounter. It is reflected in how we actively listen and effectively engage in a manner that recognizes and respects diversity and cultural differences. Cultural skill development is challenging and requires explicit awareness and practice, similar to all aspects of patient care. Consider your interview and examination techniques and how you acquired the skills necessary to determine an appropriate physical therapy diagnosis and plan of care. Cultural skill is woven into this process. One can build proficiency in cultural skill by reflecting on the impact of our biases and prejudices, learning about different cultures, maintaining awareness of global and local current events, actively engaging with others of diverse backgrounds, and utilizing emotional intelligence. Proficiency requires a growth mindset, humility, and the understanding that it is an ongoing process.

Cultural Encounters

New experiences and relationships with diverse groups of individuals throughout our careers enhance our own lives and allow us to enrich our interactions with patients and clients. Cultural encounters are an essential part of professional development. Having cultural encounters as part of your personal development plan ensures you gain opportunities to acquire knowledge and practice the skills needed to provide culturally competent patient care. Traveling, attending conferences, and participating in national and international volunteer groups are all examples of cultural encounters that impact cultural skills and enhance clinical practice.

● CULTURAL INTELLIGENCE

Another framework used to explore culturally appropriate care is cultural intelligence. Cultural intelligence, often referred to as CQ, is the ability of the individual to understand, correctly infer, function, manage, and deal with situations and characteristics of cultural diversity.[2] Cultural Intelligence (CQ) has four dimensions as described in **Table 8.2**.[3,4]

Awareness and utilization of these four dimensions reflect the facets required to function in culturally diverse environments successfully. They also integrate topics discussed in previous

TABLE 8.1. The Four Levels of Cultural Awareness

Level of Cultural Awareness	Definition
Unconscious Incompetence	Being unaware of the lack of cultural knowledge
Conscious Incompetence	Being aware of a lack of cultural knowledge
Conscious Competence	Being aware of cultural differences and possessing knowledge but not yet proficient in the application of this knowledge
Unconscious Competence	Being aware of cultural differences, possessing knowledge and proficiency in the application of this knowledge

TABLE 8.2. The Four Dimensions of Cultural Intelligence (CQ)

Dimension	Definition	Aspects
Motivational CQ	The incentive to engage appropriately in the interaction	Intrinsic Extrinsic Self-efficacy
Cognitive CQ	The knowledge of cultural rules and conventions	Cultural systems Cultural norms and values
Metacognitive CQ	The strategy to be effective in the interaction	Awareness Planning Checking
Behavioral CQ	The specific actions in a cultural encounter	Verbal Nonverbal Words and terms

TABLE 8.3. The Five Traits of Cultural Intelligence

Traits	Definition
Cultural Empathy	Connecting to the feelings, thoughts, and behaviors of those from a different culture
Cultural Flexibility	Ability to adapt to new and different situations using established personal strategies
Social Initiative	A willingness to engage with others socially
Emotional Stability	Well-developed emotional intelligence
Open-Mindedness	Reflecting on bias and potential prejudice and a willingness for acceptance of others

chapters about communication and emotional intelligence. Unlike the cultural competency model, which looks at individuals' overall development, the cultural intelligence framework focuses on each individual interaction. It allows for easy application in the clinical setting. Research suggests that individuals must leverage five traits to effectively engage in the four dimensions of cultural intelligence. The five traits are listed in **Table 8.3**.[3–5]

To summarize these concepts, cultural intelligence represents the process from thought to action within each experience with an individual or group of diverse backgrounds. Imagine each encounter as an opportunity to develop your cultural intelligence further, considering the four dimensions outlined in Table 8.2 and the traits defined in Table 8.3. Each encounter helps to strengthen your cultural competence, thus enhancing your desire, awareness, knowledge, and skills. As we add to these experiences throughout our lifetime, we gain cultural intelligence and evolve our cultural competence.

Reflection Moment

Consider the following:

1. Reflect on your desire to provide culturally competent care. Is this important to you as a professional?
2. What are the benefits of being culturally aware and acquiring cultural knowledge?
3. What does cultural skill look like in a healthcare interaction?
4. Can you think of an interaction in which the traits of cultural intelligence were effective or ineffective?

● CULTURAL QUOTIENT IN HEALTH CARE

In the health care setting, many guiding documents help clinicians understand the expectations of cultural awareness in their workplace. These documents include federal and state guidelines and regulations, organizational policies and procedures, and professional codes and practice acts. Health care clinicians must be aware of these documents and use the skills discussed above to incorporate the guidelines, regulations, and principles into everyday practice. Unfortunately, it is only possible to cover some potential guidance for cultural intelligence in a book chapter. However, there are a few documents that all physical therapists should review.

CLAS Standards

The National Culturally and Linguistically Appropriate Services (CLAS) in Health and Health Care published by the US Department of Health and Human Services Office of Minority Health include fifteen standards that "intend to advance health equity, improve quality, and help eliminate health care disparities by establishing a blueprint for health and health care organizations." These standards aid in providing organizational guidelines for cultural competence. **Table 8.4** outlines the fifteen CLAS Standards.[6]

The CLAS Standards not only guide leaders of health care organizations on patient and employee policies and procedures, but they also offer valuable information to the health care team. For example, the CLAS Standards inform team members to provide language support services to anyone whose primary language is not English. They instruct team members to include accurate demographics in the documentation. The CLAS Standards emphasize the need for health care organizations and their employees to regularly assess community needs and engage the community in determining appropriate services.

Physical Therapy Professional Guidance

The guidance for those in the physical therapy profession to adopt a CQ framework as a component of their professionalism is found in the APTA Code of Ethics for the Physical Therapist, Standards of Ethical Conduct for the Physical Therapist Assistant, and the Core Values of the Physical Therapist and Physical Therapist Assistant. As an example, Principle No. 1 of the APTA Code of Ethics states that Physical Therapists shall respect the inherent dignity and rights of all individuals. In addition, Principle No. 8 outlines physical therapists' duties to meet people's needs locally, nationally, and globally. One can only fulfill these obligations by first putting CQ as a core aspect of their professional duty. Likewise, the APTA Core Values and the Professional Behaviors for the 21st Century recognize the responsibility and skills that physical therapy professionals need to create a trusting environment with patients and society. Cultural competence is essential in building trust with those from different cultural backgrounds. These documents support the acquisition of professional skills and behaviors that effectively impact individual and societal interactions on many different levels in a culturally aware manner.

Reflection Moment

1. Take a moment and review the APTA Core Values of the Physical Therapist and Physical Therapist Assistant. List 2-3 examples of how this document integrates with cultural competence
2. Examine the Code of Ethics for Physical Therapists (Principle No. 8) and the Standards of Ethical Conduct for the Physical Therapist Assistant (Standard No. 8). What are the ways CQ connects to these components?
3. If you presented the importance of cultural intelligence in a staff meeting, how would you integrate CLAS Standards and APTA documents into the presentation?

TABLE 8.4. The National Culturally and Linguistically Appropriate Services (CLAS)

Standard	Description
Principal Standard: (1)	1. Provide effective, equitable, understandable, and respectful quality care and services that are responsive to diverse cultural health beliefs and practices, preferred languages, health literacy, and other communication needs.
Governance, Leadership, and Workforce: (2-4)	2. Advance and sustain organizational governance and leadership that promotes CLAS and health equity through policy, practices, and allocated resources. 3. Recruit, promote, and support a culturally and linguistically diverse governance, leadership, and workforce that are responsive to the population in the service area. 4. Educate and train governance, leadership, and workforce in culturally and linguistically appropriate policies and practices on an ongoing basis.
Communication and Language Assistance: (5-8)	5. Offer language assistance to individuals with limited English proficiency and/or other communication needs at no cost to facilitate timely access to all health care and services. 6. Inform all individuals of the availability of language assistance services clearly and in their preferred language, verbally and in writing. 7. Ensure the competence of individuals providing language assistance, recognizing that using untrained individuals and/or minors as interpreters should be avoided. 8. Provide easy-to-understand print and multimedia materials and signage in the languages commonly used by the populations in the service area.
Engagement, Continuous Improvement, and Accountability: (9-15)	9. Establish culturally and linguistically appropriate goals, policies, and management accountability, and infuse them throughout the organization's planning and operations. 10. Conduct ongoing assessments of the organization's CLAS-related activities and integrate CLAS-related measures into measurement and continuous quality improvement activities. 11. Collect and maintain accurate and reliable demographic data to monitor and evaluate the impact of CLAS on health equity and outcomes and to inform service delivery. 12. Conduct regular assessments of community health assets and needs and use the results to plan and implement services that respond to the cultural and linguistic diversity of populations in the service area. 13. Partner with the community to design, implement, and evaluate policies, practices, and services to ensure cultural and linguistic appropriateness. 14. Create conflict and grievance resolution processes that are culturally and linguistically appropriate to identify, prevent, and resolve conflicts or complaints. 15. Communicate the organization's progress in implementing and sustaining CLAS to all stakeholders, constituents, and the general public.

● ASSESSING CULTURAL QUOTIENT

This chapter examined the framework for cultural competence and cultural intelligence and their interconnection. We further explored the expectations of CQ in the health care industry and the profession of physical therapy. Applying standardized measures to understand your development in CQ is helpful. An assessment provides insight into your current knowledge and ability and allows you to establish goals for your professional development. **Table 8.5** briefly overviews standardized assessments for cultural competence and cultural intelligence. Explore these assessment tools and consider how you may use them to develop your CQ. Consider how these tools apply to health care team development and connect to guidance from professional standards.[2,3]

● SUMMARY

This chapter highlights how culture influences lived experiences for each of us and how we integrate our culture into our worldviews. As health care professionals, it is essential to understand the role culture plays in health care interactions and expectations of patients and the role it plays in our daily lives as health care professionals. Developing our cultural competency and applying cultural intelligence in our interaction with others requires intentional focus and evaluation for lifetime growth. Let's examine a few case studies highlighting the need for CQ in patient care and health care operations.

● CASE STUDIES

It is important to understand how CQ integrates into everyday interactions. The case studies in this section demonstrate how professionals in the field of physical therapy can use CQ to gauge professional growth. The three case studies apply cultural competence and cultural intelligence frameworks and discuss how emerging, reflective, and influencing professionals apply each framework.

TABLE 8.5. Cultural Competency Assessment Tools		
Assessment Tool	**Type of Assessment**	**Description**
Cultural Intelligence Scale (CQS)	Focuses more on cultural knowledge, not as much on attitude or behaviors	20-item assessment with four subscales: • Metacognitive • CQ Cognitive • CQ Motivation • Behavior
Cross-cultural Competency Inventory (CCCI)	Measures three aspects of cultural competence: cognitive, emotional, and behavioral	58 items in six different subscales: • Cultural adaptation • Self-presentation • Ambiguity/uncertainty tolerance • Determination • Engagement • Mission
Positive/Negative Attitude Towards Culturally Divergent People Questionnaire	Focuses on two areas of cultural interaction: attitudes and experiences of interacting with people from other cultures and attitudes toward refugees	Yes/No questionnaire focusing on experiences of an individual

CASE STUDY 1
I don't want to be a bother

Lou is a physical therapist working in an acute care hospital. He is assigned to the medical surgery floor and often works with patients immediately postoperative. Lou is aware of the impact of pain tolerance and the balance between postoperative pain and mobility needs. Lou's first patient of the day is Chan Lee, a 78-year-old male, status post a hernia repair. Mr. Lee is a Chinese-American who immigrated to the United States in his mid-30s.

Upon arriving in Mr. Lee's room, Lou notices that the patient appears uncomfortable. Mr. Lee is shifting in his bed and grimaces when moving. Lou knows from his chart review that Mr. Lee refused pain medication earlier that morning, and the nursing notes stated that his pain was bearable and that he did not want the medication. During his subjective assessment, Lou explored Mr. Lee's pain level and, again, Mr. Lee reported a pain level of 3/10 and bearable. Lou offered to follow up with the nurse for pain medication to improve Mr. Lee's pain level, but he declined.

As Lou proceeded with his evaluation and attempted to get Mr. Lee out of bed, Lou observed signs of increased pain level. Mr. Lee began sweating, breathing rapidly, and guarding movement while moving from sitting to standing. Lou assisted Mr. Lee back into bed, checked his vital signs, and revisited the pain discussion. From their conversation, Lou understands that culturally Mr. Lee felt that he should not be a burden to those around him, and as a courtesy to those around him and those more in need, he should refuse the offer of pain medication. Lou realized he needed to understand more about Mr. Lee's pain medication refusal. He decided to allow Mr. Lee to rest with a plan to return later that afternoon.

Let's examine Lou from the three levels of professional development:

 EMERGING PROFESSIONAL

As an emerging professional, Lou may lack the cultural encounters necessary to know immediately what to do. However, Lou was consciously incompetent and realized he needed more information to engage Mr. Lee in pain management best practices. Therefore, Lou used his motivational CQ to learn about cultural responses to pain and strategies for a more productive interaction with Mr. Lee during their afternoon session.

 REFLECTING PROFESSIONAL

As a reflecting professional, Lou recognized during the initial assessment that he and the nurse were approaching Mr. Lee's pain management incorrectly. Lou left the session with Mr. Lee and found the nurse to discuss a more culturally appropriate response to Mr. Lee's pain management for the afternoon session. Together the nurse and Lou developed a plan in which the nurse would offer the pain medication to Mr. Lee by informing him that using pain medication would improve the therapy session, allow for better mobility, and meet the treatment goals. Appealing to Mr. Lee's strong sense of duty and obligation would enhance his likelihood of accepting pain management and improve his mobility outcomes.

 INFLUENCING PROFESSIONAL

As an influencing clinician, Lou read Mr. Lee's chart and developed a treatment strategy for the initial evaluation. Lou decided first to have a conversation with Mr. Lee

TABLE 8.6. Case Study 1: Cultural Intelligence Framework

Dimension	Definition	Lou's Actions
Motivational CQ	The motivation to engage appropriately in the interaction	Lou understands the impact of culture on successful outcomes. Throughout his career, Lou sought out different experiences through education, working in a variety of settings, and doing volunteer work with different communities in his area.
Cognitive CQ	The knowledge of cultural rules and conventions	Lou journals about his patient encounters to learn from his personal successes and challenges; Lou integrates literature and continuing education courses about culturally competent care into his professional development plan.
Metacognitive CQ	The strategy to be effective in the interaction	Lou integrates clinical and cultural knowledge into a plan for the patient assessment before entering Mr. Lee's room and is able to employ collaborative interactions to support effective care.
Behavioral CQ	The specific actions in a cultural encounter	Lou plans his words and nonverbal cues based on prior experience and cultural knowledge.

about the need for the combination of pain medication and mobility for successful outcomes. Following the discussion, if Mr. Lee agreed to the pain medication, Lou would ask the nurse to administer the medication and plan to return in about an hour to continue the physical therapy evaluation.

As an influencing professional, Lou has unconscious competence and cultural awareness. His encounters with people from differing backgrounds, his continuing education courses, and the skill he has developed over time allow him to take a flexible approach to patient assessment. He knew that the pain medication discussion needed to be in a culturally sensitive manner to have a positive outcome. **Table 8.6** outlines Lou's interaction through the cultural intelligence framework.

CASE STUDY 2
I can speak for her

Namir works as a traveling physical therapist and recently began a new rotation in an outpatient clinic in the Washington, D.C., area. Namir has been a traveling physical therapist since graduating from DPT school three years ago. Until now, he has mainly worked in rural areas of the country and is enjoying the city and its diverse cultures. However, he realizes he has much to learn about many different cultures.

Namir's first patient on the schedule the next day is Nyala. Nyala is a 28-year-old woman who recently injured her shoulder. Nyala immigrated from Ethiopia with her husband, Kofi, and their two children a year ago. Her referral notes that she speaks very little English. Namir has not yet had experience working with language assistance programs but knows that he has to prepare for their discussion. First, Namir talks to the clinic director, Eloy, about his upcoming evaluation. Eloy reviews the Limited English Proficiency Policy for the clinic. Then, he helps Namir set up an appointment with video translation services. Excited about a new learning experience, Namir takes the time to learn how to leverage video conferencing services and researches Ethiopian culture.

The following day Nyala arrives for her appointment with her husband, Kofi. Namir enters the room and introduces himself and the video translation services. Immediately, Nyala looks a bit nervous and looks to Kofi to speak. Kofi informs Namir that he will translate for his wife and does not want a video translation service. He further states that he does not want a male therapist to work with his wife and that a woman should be assigned to work with her. Namir explains that he needs to hear this statement directly from Nyala and would happily ask another therapist to see her. However, there are only male therapists working in the center today. Kofi becomes agitated, informs Namir that this is unacceptable, and asks to reschedule Nyala's appointment when a woman can work with her.

Disappointed by this interaction and unable to redirect the situation, Namir escorts them back to the scheduling desk to reschedule the appointment and request a woman physical therapist. After they leave, Namir reflects on the situation.

Reflection Moment
Consider the following:

1. Did Namir prepare effectively for this visit? If not, what could he do differently in the future?
2. Is there a concern about the interactions between Nyala and Kofi? If so, what is Namir's responsibility?
3. How can the clinic prepare for Nyala's next visit?
4. What policies and procedures should exist to best support a positive outcome in the future?

CASE STUDY 3
The weekend schedule!

Sam recently moved from a small rural town in Pennsylvania to Pittsburgh. They were excited to start a new position as an acute care clinical director at a large urban hospital. Sam had been the clinical director in their small community hospital for the past five years, and although they loved their role, they wanted to live in a more diverse and urban location. So, when the opportunity came about, Sam took it.

They knew they would need to learn new skills about leading a team in a busy trauma center and about diverse patients and employees.

As a new manager, Sam decided their best approach was to observe the team and learn how the team functioned, what was working and what wasn't. One of the tasks Sam decided that they had to do early in their role was to understand the scheduling process for clinical rotations, time off approvals, and weekend rotations. The schedule seemed to puzzle Sam, especially the weekend schedule. In their previous role, Sam rotated the team through weekends, with staff covering both Saturday and Sunday. This rotation made it easy; you could plan out for months, knowing that every sixth weekend was your weekend. Then, if staff needed to change, they worked together to cover.

The schedule in this larger facility here was all over the place! It seemed some people never worked Saturday, and there was more staff scheduled on Sunday than Saturday, and it looked like there was no regular rotation for anyone. Sam thought to themself, "Wow, this is way too complicated! I could get an early win with the team if I made a more consistent rotation. I think I will create a mock schedule and get the team's input at our next staff meeting."

Sam was so excited, they created a simplified schedule, and it looked like the team only needed to work every sixth weekend. Sam decided they couldn't wait until the following week's staff meeting and decided to share the schedule idea with one of the team leads, Hassan. When Sam shared the schedule with Hassan, they were shocked by his response.

Hassan looked at the schedule and started to shake his head and laugh. "Sam, you can't do this," Hassan said. "Half of your team will quit, and you will end up in HR!" Sam was perplexed. "What are you talking about? This is a fair schedule."

It's not about fair," Hassan said. "It's about meeting the team's needs and understanding their life and the lives of our patients. Let's start at the beginning. Have you taken the time to learn about the lives of your team? Our team has at least four different religious holidays. Did you know that several of our staff observe Sabbat? And a good amount of our patients do also. This means staff and patients aren't available for therapy on Saturday. Our busiest weekend workdays are Sundays. If you rotate team members without having them schedule around religious holidays, you will have a mess on your hands. Our weekend schedule is a very complex and delicate balance. We work really hard to include everyone's needs. Sam, you could have made a major mistake in bringing this to the team. Here's some advice: I suggest you take time to learn about whom you supervise before changing anything."

Reflection Moment

1. At what cultural awareness level is Sam in this scenario?
2. How should Sam gain the knowledge and skills necessary to lead this team?
3. What hospital and department policies and procedures should Sam examine as guidance for inclusive employment and patient care practices?

● PROFESSIONAL DEVELOPMENT

Reflection Moment

Take a moment to reflect on your CQ, and use this time to reflect on your growth. Refer to **Table 8.7** and consider the five key elements of cultural competence and comment on your thoughts and experiences in Table 8.7.

Now, let's complete your professional strategic development plan for CQ in **Table 8.8**. This table also needs to be the width of both columns. Remember, completing this exercise at the end of each chapter helps build your overall professional development strategic plan at the end of the book.

TABLE 8.7. The Five Areas of Cultural Competence	
My Current Level of Development	
Cultural Desire	
Cultural Awareness	
Cultural Knowledge	
Cultural Skill	
Cultural Encounters	

TABLE 8.8. Professional Development Plan for CQ			
CQ Goals (No More Than 2-3)	**Tactics to Accomplish My CQ Goals**	**The Measure of Success for My CQ Goals**	**Accountability Partner: Who Will I Share My Goals with, and How Will I Check In with Them?**

References

1. Camphinha-Bacote J. *The Process of Cultural Competence in the Delivery of Healthcare Services. A Culturally Competent Model of Care.* Transcultural C.A.R.E. Association; 2003.

2. Majda A, Bodys-Cupak IE, Zalewska-Puchała J, Barzykowski K. Cultural competence and cultural intelligence of healthcare professionals providing emergency medical services. *Int J Environ Res Public Health.* 2021;18(21):11547. doi:10.3390/ijerph182111547.

3. Livermore D. *Leading with Cultural Intelligence: The New Secret to Success.* American Management Association; 2010.

4. Wang C, Shakespeare-Finch J, Dunne MP, Hou XY, Khawaja NG. How much can our universities do in the development of cultural intelligence? A cross-sectional study among health care students. *Nurse Educ Today.* 2021;103:104956. doi:10.1016/j.nedt.2021.104956.

5. van der Zee K, van Oudenhoven JP. Culture shock or challenge? The role of personality as a determinant of intercultural competence. *J Cross-Cult Psychol.* 2013;44(6):928-940. doi:10.1177/0022022113493138.

6. AHRQ. Culturally and linguistically appropriate services. https://www.ahrq.gov/sdoh/clas/index.html.

chapter 9

Social Responsibility

Chapter 1 of this book introduced professionalism on three levels—individual, interpersonal, and societal. Many of the concepts discussed in the book bring these three levels together. For example, emotional intelligence is important from an individual level and an interpersonal and societal perspective. Likewise, the cultural quotient builds from personal awareness to a societal impact. This chapter on social responsibility describes how health care professionals bring together the concepts in chapters 4 through 8 to fulfill their moral and civic duty as professionals. In this chapter, we explore concepts associated with social responsibilities, introduce the principles of social justice, discuss the role of social responsibility in health care, and apply social responsibility to case studies.

● DEFINING SOCIAL RESPONSIBILITY

When thinking about responsibilities, health care professionals often consider their responsibility for their patients, their work organizations, and even their broader profession. However, it is a stretch for each health care provider to consider the role they play each day in shaping our society. Many of us get up each day and focus on our immediate tasks, our families and friends, social groups, and the individual patients/ clients in our clinical practice. However, physical therapy professionals have a duty to look beyond those connections to our responsibility to society as a whole. Social responsibility, from the perspective of the profession of physical therapy, is the process of developing mutual trust between the profession and the public by responding to societal needs for health and wellness.[1,2] To further understand social responsibility, let's explore some underlying concepts and components influencing how professionals approach social responsibility.

Altruism

An important driver of social responsibility is the idea of altruism. Altruism is the aim or motivation to increase or benefit another's well-being and may include actions that promote the well-being of others. Although this concept and definition may appear simplistic and easy to understand, the practice of altruism can be confusing and complex. For example, is someone being altruistic if their motivations and actions benefit themselves as well as others? Let's consider a student who volunteers their time each week at a pro bono health clinic. The student is very excited to provide the services at the clinic and is demonstrating altruism through their motivations and actions. However, the student is also fulfilling a program requirement for their education by participating in the pro bono clinic, thus potentially fulfilling an egoistic, or motivation by the gratification of oneself, goal. It is important to understand that these two ideas can coexist and often do in a health care environment. Health care professionals are responsible for reflecting on and understanding the incentives behind our activities. Also, we should clearly understand our motivations and how they drive our actions. A student working at a pro bono clinic, whose only motivation is to meet the program requirements, may have a very different interaction with those receiving services from the clinic than the student whose motivations are both altruistic and egoistic goals. Health care professionals need to develop their altruism to grow their social responsibility.

Those driven to benefit others are open to opportunities to meet societal needs. As health care professionals, we may want to help others and meet societal needs, but we may need help understanding how to engage in social responsibility activities. The principles of social justice can guide us in developing a plan for social responsibility as health care professionals.

Social Justice

The origin of social justice began in the 1800s as a way to examine economic injustice created by the social class systems in Europe. This concept expanded throughout the centuries to include all human rights, including the distribution of resources, how individuals and groups are treated, and the opportunity to play a role in society.[3,4] Five principles are core to the definition of social justice and key to establishing a foundation for social responsibility. The table below defines these five principles and gives examples of how they connect to social responsibility in the health care industry.[3,4]

The principles of social justice encompass many aspects of the human experience. Therefore, they may take on different meanings for different groups of individuals. Because of the complexity and varying perceptions of social justice, it is essential to understand that barriers exist to acting in a socially responsible manner and accomplishing social justice. An example of a barrier to social justice is the idea of bias. Everyone views the world differently and therefore has some level of bias. Bias exists in different forms, and it is essential to recognize personal bias as well as the bias of others to apply social justice principles and be socially responsible. The following section explores bias and its impact on social responsibility.

Bias

The term bias refers to our favor or preference against one thing, group, or person compared to another. Bias is often seen negatively as leaving out or discriminating against something. However, our brain uses bias thousands of times daily to make many different life decisions. We use this unconscious process to determine whether the world around us is safe or pleasant. For example, you may not have enough time or knowledge to decide if an interaction may be harmful, let's say, a snake lying across a walking path; your unconscious bias may drive you to stay very clear of the snake, not knowing if this snake is venomous or not. At this moment, you don't have the time or the resources to use conscious decision-making to research and explore the potential risk the snake poses, so you rely on that unconscious bias to decide for you.[5]

Although our bias may protect us in many instances, it also drives decisions about our interactions with others in ways that cause harm.

Bias is further defined as either implicit or explicit. Implicit bias is acting on a prejudice or stereotype without intending to do so. In implicit bias, the person doesn't actively intend to act or behave in a particular manner based on prejudice or stereotype. Explicit biases are prejudice or stereotypes individuals are aware of, reflected in their actions. Both implicit and explicit biases have harmful effects and impact the professional's ability to act in a socially responsible manner.[5,6] For example, the impact of racism, sexism, and ageism in health care stems from the implicit and explicit bias of the professionals within health care systems. A research study found that when examining home exercise programs given to white and black patients with the same diagnosis, the black patients received fewer exercises in their home exercise program.[6] This study is an example of how bias may impact individuals' access to the same level of service as others. In this study, the physical therapy professionals may not consciously act in a way that provides fewer exercises to one patient over another. Still, their implicit bias may have influenced their decision-making. Clinics and health care organizations can reduce the impact of implicit bias by creating clinical pathways and best practices education to ensure a standardized approach for all patients.

Bias impacts not only individuals receiving health care services but also those working in the health care industry. For example, research points to microaggressions toward health care professionals and students based on race, gender, and age.[6-8] As professionals, we must understand the role of bias in our interactions with others and work to not only understand how bias influences our decisions but also to find ways to minimize the impact of bias. In doing so, professionals can strive to create an environment that promotes social responsibility through altruism and the principles of social justice.

Reflection Moment

Consider your experience in your current professional/student role and perhaps as a patient:

1. Have you experienced discrimination based on another's bias? How did that affect you?
2. Consider your own bias; how might it influence your professional development?
3. What strategies might you use to recognize your bias and minimize the impact on your professional development?
4. Choose a principle of social justice from **Table 9.1**. How might your actions based on that principle of social justice change as you develop your professionalism?

Discuss from an emerging, reflecting, and influencing professional's perspective.

● SOCIAL RESPONSIBILITY IN HEALTH CARE

From the examples above, we can see many aspects of social responsibility in health care. Social responsibility starts with each of us doing our part and working collectively to impact society. Advocacy is a powerful example of how social responsibility works in health care. From an individual level, we may advocate for the unique needs of our patients. This may include advocating for access to services, equitable care, or being our patients' voices. Also, as individuals, we may advocate for our profession and services. This advocacy could exist at an organizational level by advocating for budgetary resources to gain access to better equipment for patient care or at a professional level by visiting members of Congress to discuss policy that impacts our profession and our patients. As a collective, health care organizations and professionals advocate and gain justice for patients and communities. The policy agenda of professional organizations such as the APTA is an example of their social responsibility to their members and the patients/clients they serve. **Table 9.2** provides examples of the APTA policy agenda and its connection to social responsibility.

The APTA Public Policy Priorities build on guidance from the APTA core documents. As professionals, having these core documents as a resource helps us understand the expectations of our profession and how we should strive to meet the needs of society. **Table 9.3** summarizes important aspects of the guiding documents and how they relate to our role in social responsibility.

Integrating the principles of social justice and altruism, striving to reduce the impact of bias in health care, and applying the core tenants of social responsibility as defined by our

TABLE 9.1. Principles of Social Justice

	Definition	Social Responsibility Examples in Health Care
Access	The ability to obtain the necessary resource. Examples include food, shelter, education, and health care.	A mobile health clinic that travels to rural areas to provide health screening
Equity	Providing individual support needed to achieve goals. This is NOT equality, which is giving everyone the same resources.	Providing a written home exercise program to one person but providing a voice-recorded home and exercise program for another person who has a visual impairment
Diversity	Acknowledging that differences exist between individuals and groups; embracing these differences, consideration of the difference in policy, planning, and actions	Providing a prayer and meditation room in a hospital with an altar and floor mat to accommodate different prayer and meditation needs
Participation	Providing a platform and opportunity for every individual to have their voice heard as part of decision and policy-making	Conducting community research to best understand community needs before developing a health clinic
Human Rights	The right of each person to have freedoms such as free speech, the ability to vote for elected officials, and the right to a fair trial	Providing patient advocates to support patients in voicing concerns regarding their care

TABLE 9.2. Examples of APTA Public Policy Goals

Public Policy	Aspects of Social Responsibility
Improve patient outcomes by eliminating barriers to health care services	Access Equity Human Rights
Enact policies that empower all people, regardless of where they are born, live, learn, work, play, worship, and age, to live healthy and independent lives	Altruism Equity Diversity Human Rights
Improve patient outcomes and patient satisfaction by improving health services delivery	Access Participation
Prioritize research and clinical innovation to advance the science, effectiveness, and efficacy of physical therapist evaluation and management to optimize patient health, well-being, and recovery	Access Diversity Equity

Adapted from APTA Public Policy Priorities 2021-2022[9]

professional organizations are ways physical therapy professionals act in a socially responsible manner. However, physical therapy professionals can move beyond everyday actions to transform society. The following section discusses ways physical therapy professionals can promote social responsibility in our communities.

● PROMOTING SOCIAL RESPONSIBILITY IN OUR COMMUNITIES

"Transforming society through optimizing human movement to improve the human experience" is a vision that guides physical therapy professionals to move beyond their role in the clinical setting into the community.[11] Community service, service learning, and pro bono clinics are all examples of ways physical therapy professionals strive to achieve this vision. Community service can mean service to your profession through volunteering in your professional organization, service to your community through such activities as volunteering at local health fairs, or

TABLE 9.3. Social Responsibility from the APTA Guiding Documents

Core Document	Statement
Vision Statement	Transforming society by optimizing movement to improve the human experience.
Core Values for the Physical Therapist and Physical Therapist Assistant	**Social responsibility** is the promotion of a mutual trust between the profession and the larger public that necessitates responding to societal needs for health and wellness.
Code of Ethics for the Physical Therapist	**Principle No. 5** Physical therapists shall fulfill their legal and professional obligations. **Principle No. 8** Physical therapists shall participate in efforts to meet the health needs of people locally, nationally, or globally.
Standards of Ethical Conduct for the Physical Therapist Assistant	**Standard No. 5** Physical therapist assistants shall fulfill their legal and ethical obligations. **Standard No. 8** Physical therapist assistants shall participate in efforts to meet the health needs of people locally, nationally, or globally.

Adapted from APTA Guiding Documents[1,2,10]

even service to our global society through health care mission trips. When students participate in experiential learning activities where they apply academic knowledge to meet the community's needs, they act in a socially responsible manner through service learning. Other examples of service are participating in community action research, advocacy, and pro bono services. As a physical therapy professional, you can play an essential role in achieving the profession's vision.

Reflection Moment

1. Consider your current role. Do you consider yourself socially responsible? If yes, provide some examples of how you act in a socially responsible manner through your daily activities.
2. Are you socially responsible beyond your role with patients and clients? List ways you participate in community service, advocacy, service learning, or pro bono activities.
3. Consider our vision statement. In what ways can physical therapy professionals transform society?

● SUMMARY

In this chapter, we explored concepts associated with social responsibilities, introduced the principles of social justice, examined the role of social responsibility within health care, and discussed ways for physical therapy professionals to incorporate social responsibility into daily clinical practice and within their communities. Understanding how we apply social responsibility in clinical settings and our communities is important. The following section discusses four case studies that demonstrate different ways physical therapy professionals act in a socially responsible manner and provides guiding questions for additional reflection.

CASE STUDY 1
Community service matters to me

Ryder grew up in a family who valued community service. Ryder was involved in community activities with his parents from a young age. He always loved these experiences. So, when Ryder was accepted into a physical therapist assistant program, he knew he wanted to use his skills as a PTA to give back to the community. In his educational experience, he gained an understanding of the APTA Core Values and the role of social responsibility in his profession. In his second year of PTA school, Ryder decided it was time to plan ways to give back by using his skills as a PTA. The only problem was that he wasn't sure what to do next. The PTA program he attended had some brief volunteer activities for students, but it wasn't to the extent that Ryder wanted. Ryder decided to go to his faculty advisor to discuss what he needed to have in place to start his community service as a PTA.

Consider a potential conversation between Ryder and his faculty advisor:

1. If you were Ryder's faculty advisor, what steps might you encourage him to take as a student and a new graduate?
2. What guiding documents does Ryder need to use in establishing his plan, and why are these documents important?
3. What regulations, laws, and other areas might Ryder need to consider?
4. What principles of social justice is Ryder fulfilling in his desire to participate in community service?

CASE STUDY 2
Pronouns

Alexa recently graduated from physical therapy school and planned to interview for a job at a local hospital. Alexa was a bit nervous about the interview. They grew up in a small midwestern town and knew some of the staff at the hospital. Alexa had recently changed their name from Alex to Alexa and began using they/them pronouns. Alexa's family and friends were very supportive of their nonbinary identity. However, Alexa was nervous about how their identity would be accepted in the work environment and by members of the community who knew them as Alex.

When Alexa began the application process, they were happy to see their pronouns as an option on the application. Alexa decided to wear their favorite skirt and jacket on the day of the interview. Although they felt most comfortable in this outfit, they knew that they might interact with members of their community who might question their choice of clothing. Alexa's interview consisted of meeting with the Director of Rehabilitation, members of the physical therapy team, and the human resource representative. Alexa was pleasantly surprised when everyone used their current pronouns and treated them in a warm and welcoming manner. Alexa even interacted with a nursing supervisor, Nancy, who knew their parents. Nancy used Alexa's correct name and pronouns and complemented Alexa on their professional attire. After the interview day, Alexa was confident that they wanted to work at the hospital.

Consider this case study:

1. What principles of social justice were the team members at the hospital following?
2. How might this interaction impact Alexa as an emerging professional?
3. What level of professionalism is Nancy demonstrating? Support your thoughts.
4. What implicit bias could have negatively impacted this interaction?
5. What role did organizational responsibility and process play in this interaction?

CASE STUDY 3
She never does the home exercise program

Maria just started as a physical therapist in the only pediatric clinic in rural Arkansas. She moved after she married her husband, who was from the area. Although Maria loved her job in the children's hospital where she lived before getting married, she was confident she could make an impact in her new role in this rural region. She was amazed at how invested the clinic seemed in the community and that parents from over an hour away would bring their children to the clinic.

During her first month, Maria bonded with several children and their families. She liked getting to know members of the community. However, there was one mom, Trisha, who, unfortunately, was frustrating Maria. In every session, Trisha was involved and acted like she wanted to do what was best for her child. However, when she returned for subsequent sessions, she hadn't filled out the activity log for her child and didn't seem like she followed any of the detailed instructions Maria had provided. When Maria questioned her, she always seemed to have an excuse. Maria shared this frustration with a more senior coworker, Linda, who had become an informal mentor to Maria.

Linda listened intently to Maria's concerns and frustrations and then asked a critical question: "Are you sure that Trisha can read?" Maria was shocked by this question. "Well, I am sure she can read. She signed the initial paperwork, I saw her review it, and she had no questions about it." Linda paused and asked Maria, "Are you sure she can read?" Maria took some time to reflect on the question. Had she missed the signs that Trisha couldn't read and therefore had not been adequately preparing her to work with her child? After reflecting, Maria realized that Trisha always seemed to agree with everything Maria reviewed and never had any questions. She also quickly changed the subject if Maria asked to clarify anything by reading.

Maria realized she missed an important factor in providing the best care for her patient. She did not want to impose additional stress on Trisha and wasn't sure of the next steps.

Consider the following:

1. What do you think Maria should do next?
2. How can Maria move forward and create a positive outcome for Trisha and her child?
3. What is Linda's professionalism level? Support your thoughts then use **Table 9.4** to consider.
4. How might you determine the health literacy of your patients?
5. What policies and procedures should exist to support patients and families with low literacy and health literacy?

6. What principles of social justice are at play in this case study?

CASE STUDY 4
I am an advocate

Amida never described herself as an advocate. She had no problem speaking up when a patient needed something or a barrier existed for a patient. However, Amida felt that this is what she should do as a physical therapist assistant. Lately, however, Amida grew frustrated with the reimbursement for physical therapist assistants and how it impacted which patients she could work with and what services she could provide. This was especially frustrating when all of her training and continuing education in advanced therapeutic interventions didn't seem to matter. Amida has prided herself in participating in clinical education annually and applying the newest evidence-informed skills in her sessions. However, it seemed like her twelve years of experience and clinical excellence didn't matter. Amida voiced her frustration to the clinic director Mya one day. Mya wholeheartedly agreed and suggested that Amida reach out to her state chapter and see how she could get more involved in the state chapter's advocacy committee.

Although it seemed daunting, Amida decided that it was in the best interest of her patients that she pursued advocacy work. Over the next few months, Amida gained information about recent changes in regulations and reimbursement, reached out to her state chapter, and was pleasantly surprised by how easy it was for her to get involved in the advocacy committee. So, now here she was, only a few months after that conversation, headed to Washington, D.C. to participate in Advocacy Day. Amida was nervous but knew she needed to have her voice heard. She really couldn't believe that it was so easy to get involved and start making an impact on her patients and her profession.

Consider this case study:

1. At what level of professionalism is Amida? Support your thoughts.
2. What social justice principles is Amida applying?
3. How might Amida continue to expand her role in social responsibility?
4. What impact might Amida make on patient care and the profession of physical therapy?

TABLE 9.4. Case Study 3—Your Impact on Social Justice	
Ways I can Impact Social Justice:	
Access	
Equity	
Diversity	
Participation	
Human Rights	

TABLE 9.5. Professional Development Plan for Social Responsibility

Social Responsibility Goals (No More Than 2-3)	Tactics to Accomplish My Social Responsibility Goals	The Measure of Success for My Social Responsibility Goals	Accountability Partner: Who Will I Share My Goals with, and How Will I Check In with Them?

PROFESSIONAL DEVELOPMENT

Reflection Moment

Take a moment to reflect on social responsibility and use this time to reflect on your current level and areas of growth. Then, consider the five principles of social justice and how you might act in a socially responsible manner to create a more just health care system.

Now, let's complete your professional strategic development plan for social responsibility using **Table 9.5**. Remember, completing the plan in each chapter helps build your overall professional development strategic plan at the end of the book.

References

1. Swisher LL, Hiller P, for the APTA Task Force to revise the core ethics documents. The revised APTA code of ethics for the physical therapist and standards of ethical conduct for the physical therapist assistant: theory, purpose, process, and significance. *Phys Ther.* 2010;90(5):803-824. doi:10.2522/ptj.20090373.
2. Core values for physical therapist and physical therapist assistant HOD P09-21-21-09. Published online December 14, 2021. https://www.apta.org/apta-and-you/leadership-and-governance/policies/core-values-for-the-physical-therapist-and-physical-therapist-assistant. Accessed April 10, 2022.
3. Soken-Huberty E. Four principles of social justice. http://www.humanrightscareers.com/issues/four-principles-of-social-justice/.
4. Fuhriman T. 2017.04. Social equity: adaptation of social justice from law and policy to American public administration [4133]. 2017;28:298.
5. Zarn Urankar M, Wolfe GS, Pepper JD. Training implicit bias and awareness of the impact of systemic racism on health: a preliminary study of second-year optometry students. *Optom Educ.* 2022;47(3):32-42.
6. Cavanaugh AM, Rauh MJ. Does patient race affect physical therapy treatment recommendations? *J Racial Ethn Health Disparities.* 2021;8(6):1377-1384. doi:10.1007/s40615-020-00899-0.
7. Bissell BD, Johnston JP, Smith RR, et al. Gender inequity and sexual harassment in the pharmacy profession: evidence and call to action. *Am J Health Syst Pharm.* 2021;78(22):2059-2076.
8. Dickson JJ. Supporting a generationally diverse workforce: considerations for aging providers in the US healthcare system. *J Best Pract Health Prof Divers Educ Res Policy.* 2015;8(2):1071-1086.
9. American Physical Therapy Association 2021-2022 public policy priorities. Published online February 22, 2021. https://www.apta.org/advocacy/issues/apta-public-policy-priorities.
10. Standards of ethical conduct for the physical therapist assistant HOD Soc-20-31-26. Published online 8/12/2020. https://www.apta.org/apta-and-you/leadership-and-governance/policies/standards-of-ethical-conduct-for-the-physical-therapist-assistant. Accessed February 5, 2023.
11. APTA vision, mission, and strategic plan. https://www.apta.org/apta-and-you/leadership-and-governance/vision-mission-and-strategic-plan.

chapter 10

Management of Self through Lifelong Learning

This book focuses on skills that aid in personal and professional development. While these skills, communication, emotional intelligence, accountability, awareness of culture, and social responsibility, play a role in self-management, they do not paint the complete picture. This chapter explores the definition of self-management and discusses the role of self-efficacies, lifelong learning, efficient use of time and resources, and networking in professional self-management. When reading this chapter, consider how the concepts presented in previous chapters play a role in self-regulation and personal and professional growth.

In a professional setting, self-management consists of developing strategies that enhance effectiveness in the day-to-day functions of professional roles and responsibilities.[1,2] Self-management strategies build on a foundation of self-efficacy, or a belief in your abilities to perform your professional roles and responsibilities. From the foundation of self-efficacy, professionals need to develop a toolbox of skills to increase effectiveness. Essential skills include lifelong learning, wise use of time and resources, and creating a solid network of individuals who support your professional growth. Let's examine self-efficacy and these skills in more detail.[1,2]

● DEFINING SELF-EFFICACY

Self-efficacy is an individual's judgment of their ability to use resources available to complete a task. In other words, self-efficacy can be thought of as believing in their abilities.[1] As we learn new skills, our self-efficacy and belief in self-ability grow. This growth happens through a few different approaches. First, we practice the skill. And as we grow in skill mastery, our belief that we can consistently perform the skill grows. We also gain self-efficacy when others provide verbal persuasion and positive

reinforcement of skill achievement. Self-efficacy growth occurs with verbal feedback from others and the demonstration of effective skill performance in action, referred to as social modeling. Having cheerleaders while learning a skill and observing those we look up to or trust to complete the skill are powerful reinforcements to self-efficacy. This is why individuals who seek out mentors and coaches to build strong social networks often develop a strong sense of personal ability to achieve goals. In addition to external input, our mental and emotional states and our ability to imagine our accomplishments help build our self-efficacy. Just the ability to imagine that we can accomplish something and being relaxed and focused on the task improves our belief that we can gain a new skill. All of these factors align to set one up for successful skill attainment. As you gain new skills as a professional, your self-efficacy to manage your role's day-to-day functions increases. Each new skill improves your confidence to take on new and different roles and responsibilities and expand your professional abilities. Let's take a moment to consider your development of professional self-efficacy.[1,2]

Reflection Moment

Consider your educational or early professional journey and reflect on when you learned a new skill, such as a manual technique or correct transfer skills.

1. Who provided verbal persuasion that you could perform the skill? In what ways did they do so?
2. Did you leverage social modeling to accomplish the skill? If so, who was your mentor?
3. How did your emotional and mental state impact your ability to learn that skill?
4. Was there a time when your emotional and mental state limited your ability to gain a new skill?

5. Did you mentally practice the skill or go over it in your head? If so, how did that help you develop your skill level?

● LIFELONG LEARNING

Lifelong learners have an internal drive to pursue knowledge, develop new skills, and take on new challenges. Lifelong learners are curious and use their growth mindset to seek new knowledge and activities. Lifelong education is essential for professional growth and requires a strategic plan to facilitate learning throughout your career.[3] The following section provides an overview of some of these strategies:

1. **Set goals**. Throughout this book, we provided opportunities to set professional goals and establish foundational lifelong learning skills. It is important to examine and set new goals regularly. This habit helps to keep you focused on learning and growth.
2. **Read.** We read a lot when we are in school. It is easy to lose the habit of reading professionally or personally when no longer in an environment where it is required. However, professional development requires us to gain new knowledge through exploring contemporary literature, staying up to date on trends in our industry, and reviewing our practice to ensure we remain current and effective. Creating a professional reading habit early in your career promotes lifelong learning and the ability to stay current in your profession.
3. **Embrace new experiences.** Although habit and routine are a great way to ensure progress toward goals, you also want to get out of your comfort zone and experience new opportunities. These new opportunities challenge your brain and reinforce the process of creating self-efficacy. When thinking about new experiences, it is essential to consider both personal and professional experiences. A mistake people often make is that they believe it has to be a significant experience to have an impact. Different experiences in all shapes and sizes matter. For example, trying a new type of food, changing your workout routine, or implementing a new treatment approach in your practice are all new experiences that add to lifelong learning.
4. **Learn from failure.** Learning from failure incorporates concepts covered in previous chapters, such as emotional intelligence, grit, and accountability. Taking the time to examine failures and understand your role in what went wrong is a valuable learning tool. You can enhance your professional development by having an organized process to review actions and events that didn't go as planned. Reflection on situations and determining learning opportunities gained from failure provide meaningful learning objectives and create lasting impressions.
5. **Reflect on your learning.** Reflection is an ongoing theme in this book. Life is busy, and it is easy to keep moving forward without looking back. Instead, considering what we learned, how we learned best, and the next steps to scaffold learning opportunities are necessary for lifelong learning. Learning reflection helps with the first item discussed in lifelong learning, setting goals. With reflection, goals may align with learning needs. Journaling and keeping reflections in one

place where you can reference back through time provides an optimal environment for lifelong learning. It gives insight into how goals and actions help you progress, and seeing progress over time motivates you.

As you can see, lifelong learning doesn't just happen. It requires a purposeful approach, solid habits, and grit for continued professional development. Take a moment to reflect on your current approach to lifelong learning.

Reflection Moment
Consider the following questions:

1. Do I set goals for myself? If so, do I regularly re-evaluate my goals and update them?
2. How can I plan to incorporate goal-setting into my professional development?
3. Do I make a point to read new literature and industry materials to stay current on changes in my profession?

- If you answered yes, consider where you receive your professional resources. Consider ways to expand your learning opportunities through other resources.
- If you answered no, consider a goal to add at least one new professional article or resource monthly to create a reading habit for professional development.

4. Reflect on new experiences. How have they created learning opportunities and new ways of thinking?
5. Consider a time that you failed. Did you use an organized approach to reflecting on that failure? How did that failure shape your future? What did you learn from it?

● EFFICIENT USE OF TIME AND RESOURCES

Time is valuable, and resources in health care, such as patient care supplies and equipment, are limited. When we consider self-management as professionals, using time and resources wisely are valuable skills. However, these skills are something that takes practice and knowledge to develop. A new professional should consider strategies to develop these skills and regularly evaluate their effectiveness in utilizing their time and the available resources. Let's look closer at ways to enhance time management and resource utilization.

Time Management
One of the critical considerations for time management is to know yourself. In Chapter 4, we discussed the DISC behavioral styles. Using assessments such as the DISC to understand your unique behaviors is one way to begin understanding some time management strategies that help you with daily efficiency. For example, we gain energy from doing things that come easily to us, while more challenging things can drain our energy. If you tend to focus better in the early part of the day and feel less focused in the later afternoon, the performance of challenging tasks in the earlier part of the day will improve your efficiency. Considering DISC behavioral styles, if you are more people-oriented, such as the "I" or "S" styles, doing activities that are very task and detailed-oriented in the morning is a more

efficient use of your time.[4] Understanding the specific duties of your profession and connecting them to your style is just one way to improve your time management. Understanding the specific professional duties and their required time allocations is another crucial step towards better time management skills. For example, a letter of medical necessity may require research and time to outline the letter before writing. Realizing that this time is necessary and planning for that during your week is a step toward good time management, leading to improved professional self-management. This process, called time blocking, clears space in your schedule for actions requiring more focused thought and concentration. Efficient professionals often time block weekly for projects and consider the necessary time and the best time of the day to do specific tasks.

Resource Utilization

Health care professionals must think critically about necessary resources for optimal patient/client outcomes. These resources must meet the needs of the patient/client and fit within the constraints of available payment coverage, regulatory guidance, and availability in that specific health care setting. Health care professionals must rely on their lifelong learning strategies to understand the changing environment for specific patient needs, payment structures, and regulatory guidelines to ensure the best path forward for patient/client services. As professionals develop lifelong learning skills and understand the best resources for supporting clinical, payment, and regulatory knowledge, they develop efficient self-management skills in resource utilization. Reflecting on lifelong learning, health care professionals should consider what specific tasks improve their abilities to effectively utilize available resources for each patient/client. Take a moment to reflect on your current time management and resource utilization skills.

Reflection Moment

1. Think about last week. Reflect on a day that you used your time most efficiently.
2. What strategies did you use that day? What type of tasks did you do at what time of the day? How did you stay focused on the activities you completed?
3. Now consider a day you used your time least efficiently. What was your emotional state that day? What task did you attempt to complete at what time of the day? Did you have a plan when you started that day? If so, what changed the plan?
4. What resources do you use to understand patient/client management changes? How do you learn about new payment and regulatory changes?
5. If you are a physical therapy student, how will you stay current in patient/client management, payment, and regulatory changes?

● BUILDING YOUR NETWORK

Those around us play an essential role in shaping us. This is true in both personal and professional life. To grow professionally, we need to be purposeful about connecting to and understanding the unique roles each individual plays in our development.

In Chapter 11, we will discuss the roles of mentors and coaches. Although these roles are critical in our professional development, we must consider our overall professional network and how it impacts our careers. Through networking, we access new ideas, efficiencies, and resources to provide optimal care to our patients/clients and build our careers.

One way to think about your network is to consider the support required for all your different needs as a professional. Who in your current network supports those needs, and what additional support is necessary? **Figure 10.1** demonstrates a professional network in which other individuals have unique roles in professional growth. We should surround ourselves with others who support and guide our paths and allow us to see situations with a growth mindset. For example, you may have an individual who helps navigate the political work environment. This person may help you understand who has specific influences in the workplace. You may have another person who enables you to understand your emotional and logical view of a situation and whom you rely on to push back when you are uncompromising about a task. It is essential to reflect on who these people are in your network and whether there are areas where you need to add mentors or coaches. It is also crucial to understand the roles you play in the professional networks of others and how these interactions help to support professional growth and lifelong learning.

Reflection Moment

Consider your current environment.

1. Who is in your network? What roles do they play?
2. In what area do you need additional support?
3. What roles do you play in other's networks? What examples support that role?

Ways to Build Your Network

As you grow professionally, you should develop strategies to build your network. Like other aspects of professional development, building your professional network is not something you want to leave to chance. A plan to develop your network ensures

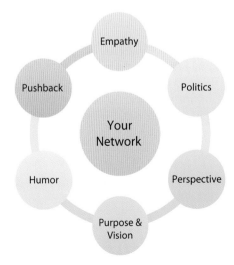

FIGURE 10.1. Professional Network.

TABLE 10.1. Creating Opportunities for Networking	
Stay Connected to Your University	This connection keeps you connected to those who graduated from the program and new graduates and faculty. This is also a great way to stay current in clinical practice. Consider volunteering as a lab assistant or guest lecturer.
Join Professional Organizations	Professional organizations provide many different levels of networking, from clinical mentors to career development and professional advocacy opportunities.
Volunteer for Committees and Task Forces within Your Organization	This is a great way to build interprofessional networks and grow organizational, political, and leadership influence.
Attend Conferences and Educational Events	Educational events provide opportunities to gain knowledge and give you time and space to meet others with similar interests and experiences. Planning on meeting at least one new colleague at every educational event is a simple and fun way to build your professional network.
Introduce Yourself	This seems simple, yet we often don't do this. Introducing yourself to new people can seem intimidating. But practicing these skills and watching others gives you self-efficacy in this vital strategy. Starting on social media in networking groups is a safe and easy way to initiate this practice and then build to introducing yourself at community and professional events.
Build Connections at all Levels	Be purposeful about having connections at all levels of organizations and your profession. Reach out to peers, those you can mentor such as students and new graduates, and those in leadership or with subject matter expertise.

that you have access to those who help you grow and can expose you to new knowledge and opportunities. **Table 10.1** outlines some ways to create networking opportunities.

● SELF-MANAGEMENT: WHY IT MATTERS IN HEALTH CARE

This chapter discusses many factors contributing to self-management. Focusing on these areas improves your ability to work more efficiently and have a better work experience. However, in the health care industry, these factors also play a crucial role in the patient experience and overall health outcomes. Patient satisfaction is a measure that health care organizations and payors utilize when determining the impact of health care services. Professional behaviors such as communication, emotional intelligence, and effective use of time and resources play a role in a patient's overall perception of the quality of care. Research has shown that these factors often influence patients' perception of the quality of their care and the overall outcome more so than the clinician's expertise and the treatment intervention type.[5-7] An example of how efficient use of time and resources impacts health care is the measure of wait time for services. Research on patient satisfaction indicates that wait time plays a role in how patients perceive the quality of their care and how satisfied they are with the services.[5,6,8] A clinician's ability to stay on schedule and organize their day influences how patients feel about the quality of care. As another example, in a study examining patient satisfaction with physical therapy services, factors such as wait time had more of an impact than the type and duration of treatment.[8]

Physical therapy professionals can play a direct role in improving patient outcomes and satisfaction in our health care system. There are many examples of the role of physical therapy in effectively using resources. For example, direct access to physical therapy reduces the need for an initial physician visit, improves overall access to services, and has shown favorable outcomes. This is seen in the outpatient setting and the use of emergency department access to physical therapy. A study examining emergency department physical therapy found that patients triaged directly to a physical therapist for musculoskeletal injuries improved patient outcomes and increased the emergency department's overall efficiency.[9]

Payors, such as insurance companies and Medicare, look for ways to reduce costs and improve patient outcomes by efficiently using resources within the health care system. Models such as value-based care, which links payment directly to patient outcomes and efficient and effective care, reward health care providers who utilize resources best while creating positive patient outcomes. Team members who effectively use resources and recognize ways to increase efficiency in processes and workflow within a health care organization can impact the overall success of a health care organization.[10,11]

Effective use of time and resources is just one example of how physical therapy professionals' self-management skills can impact health care delivery. In **Table 10.2**, let's take a moment to reflect on other ways physical therapy professionals with well-developed self-management skills can influence health care delivery. Considering patient satisfaction, patient outcomes, and the impact of reimbursement, consider ways that physical therapy professionals can leverage self-efficacy, lifelong learning, and networking through each level of professional development.

TABLE 10.2. Lifelong Professional Development			
	Emerging	Reflecting	Influencing
Self-efficacy			
Lifelong Learning			
Networking			

SUMMARY

This chapter discusses key components of self-management. It emphasizes how physical therapy professionals can build these skills to enhance their knowledge, skills, and behaviors while improving patient outcomes, satisfaction, and health care delivery. Physical therapy professionals should seek experiences and opportunities to enhance learning and engage with others who model clinical and professional skills. Professionals at all levels should strive to grow their network to connect with others who enhance their professional development.

CASE STUDIES

Understanding the relationship between self-management and improvement in health care delivery is vital to successful career development. In this section, we examine four case scenarios focusing on components of self-management. When reviewing the case examples, consider how different skills evolve when professionals move from emerging to reflecting to influencing levels of professionalism.

CASE STUDY 1
School is over! No more reading for me!

Garrett can't wait! They are starting their last clinical affiliation in their DPT program. A "normal" life of working a job and having all their free time to do what they want is just around the corner. No more late-night studying and hours of reading and researching. During their first week of clinical, they notice their clinical instructor, Brice, carrying a stack of research articles out to his car as they leave for the day. This surprises Garrett, and they ask Brice if they are working on getting a certification or returning to school. Brice smiles and responds, "Oh no, Garrett, I read several research articles each month to ensure I stay current with my clinical skills. It's a goal I set for myself when I started working." Garrett was a bit surprised; they had never talked to prior clinical instructors about how much they read or did outside their job. Sure, they knew professionals attended continuing education to keep their license current, and some decided to get additional certifications. Still, they never considered the need to read research for the rest of their career.

The next day at the clinic, Garrett observed Brice walk a patient through a new exercise program. Garrett was unfamiliar with what Brice was doing, so they asked Brice about the exercise program after the session. Brice stated, "Well, you know all that reading I did the other day… guess where I got this new idea!" Brice could tell that Garrett was still unsure about this commitment to lifelong learning. So, he suggested they talk more about lifelong learning and how it could be a fun and rewarding part of their career. Begrudgingly, Garrett agreed to discuss lifelong learning plans.

Reflection Moment

As an influencing professional, Brice has the opportunity to make a positive impact on Garrett's future.

1. What strategies should Brice suggest to Garrett to make lifelong learning a fun and rewarding part of their career development?

2. What feedback might Brice give Garrett's school about student perception of lifelong learning?

CASE STUDY 2
Sam must have an easier caseload!

Mike has been working as a physical therapist assistant in acute care for the past five years, and although he loved the fast pace of the hospital, he wanted to see patients for more than a few sessions in order to see long-term outcomes. So, when a home health PTA position within his health system opened, he jumped at the opportunity. The home health agency assigned Sam, a physical therapist assistant who has worked in home health for the past seven years, as Mike's preceptor. Sam and Mike hit it off immediately, and Mike enjoyed working with the patients in their home environment. Mike was also very impressed with how Sam engaged with the patients, completed the treatment plan, and walked out of the house with all of the documentation finished. This home health environment was great! After several weeks of precepting, Mike was confident he was ready to go it alone. In just a few short weeks, Mike was on the road seeing a full caseload, but things weren't as smooth as they appeared with Sam. Mike often ran behind schedule, had to spend time moving things around, and found that much of his documentation was left until he got home. He didn't understand. Sam had made everything look easy. Mike wondered if Sam had an easier caseload without as many patients with complex needs and obstacles. Mike reached out to Sam to discuss his frustration. After explaining his challenges, Sam suggested they consider Mike's time management and resource utilization. Sam explained that when he first started in home health, he struggled with organizing his day and patient schedule, and he found that he was always running back to the office for supplies or equipment. Mike felt relieved. These were the same struggles he was facing. And he began to see that the time and resource management techniques he had used in acute care didn't serve him well in the home health setting. Mike decided to spend a little more time with Sam and pay attention to how he organized his time and resources.

Reflection Moment

1. Discuss how Sam displayed self-efficacy as a reflecting professional in this scenario.
2. How is Sam helping Mike build self-efficacy?
3. What networking role is Sam fulfilling for Mike in this scenario?
4. Describe some potential time management techniques that Mike could use to increase his efficiency

CASE STUDY 3
Challenges of a traveling physical therapist in a rural clinic

Corie decided to work as a traveling physical therapist after the first year of her career. She knew she would have to be independent in her role and might find herself in challenging environments. She decided that before starting her journey, she would ensure she had a network of people to contact for questions and advice. She also researched the practice act in the state where she would be employed, so she knew her guidelines for supervision and clinical practice. With all of her preparation, Corie still had many challenges in her new role. The clinic she was assigned was in a rural area where she was the only physical therapist within a 50-mile radius. The small clinic had minimal equipment, one rehab tech, and a part-time office person. It was adjacent to a federal health clinic, her largest referral source. Many patients had limited insurance coverage for physical therapy and limited resources for medical supplies and transportation to physical therapy. Although Corie felt confident in her clinical skills and knew she could reach out to colleagues with clinical questions, she hadn't put a strategy in place to deal with the demands of a minimally staffed and supplied clinic and patients with such limited resources. Corie realized she would need to understand how to most efficiently use her resources and find creative ways to get necessary resources for her clinic and patients. This was a real challenge, but Corie was up to it!

Reflection Moment

Consider the areas Corie needs to manage and develop resources.

1. What organizations and sources might Corie use to find resources for her clinic?
2. What strategies might Corie use to maximize her limited clinic resources?
3. How would Corie best organize the clinic staffing resources to improve patient care and maintain appropriate supervision of support staff?
4. As an emerging professional, how can Corie leverage her network to improve her use of clinic resources and leverage patients' resources to meet their needs?

CASE STUDY 4
Network, network, network!

Serina graduated from a physical therapist assistant program three years ago and began working at a local hospital.

During her first year, she took an opportunity to join a task force focused on improving patient transportation between departments. Serina enjoyed her experience on the task force and found that others appreciated her insight as a new professional. This experience led Serina to consider leadership roles in her future. Serina knew that building her network would help her achieve this goal, but she wasn't sure what steps to take to establish her support structure. Luckily, Serina maintained a connection with the hospital administrator, Madeline, who chaired the task force. So, Serina decided to reach out to Madeline for guidance.

Reflection Moment

As an emerging professional, reaching out to Madeline is an important step for Serina; she knows she needs a plan of action for the conversation. Develop Serina's plan of action for her meeting with Madeline and consider the following:

1. What questions should she ask Madeline?
2. What time expectations should Serina have of Madeline?
3. What questions should Serina be prepared to answer?

Now take a moment to consider Madeline as a reflective or influencing professional:

1. What expectations should she have of Serina?
2. What questions might she ask Serina?
3. How can she best support Serina in her professional development?

● PROFESSIONAL DEVELOPMENT

Take a moment to reflect on your self-management skills. Use **Table 10.3** to consider the five areas of self-management and examine your current level of development.

Now, let's complete your professional strategic development plan for self-management using **Table 10.4**. Remember, completing the plan in each chapter helps build your overall professional development strategic plan at the end of the book.

TABLE 10.3. Five Areas of Self-Management	
My Current Level of Development	
Self-efficacy	
Lifelong Learning	
Time Management	
Resource Utilization	
Networking	

TABLE 10.4. Professional Development Plan for Self-Management			
Self-Management Goals (No More Than 2-3)	**Tactics to Accomplish My Self-Management Goals**	**Measure of Success for My Self-Management Goals**	**Accountability Partner: Who Will I Share My Goals with, and How Will I Check In with Them?**

References

1. Suess J. Power to the people: Why self-management is important. Published September 14, 2015. https://er.educause.edu/blogs/2015/9/power-to-the-people-why-self-management-is-important#:~:text=At%20the%20core%20of%20self,and%20nurturing%20your%20personal%20network.

2. Amamou S, Vandercleyen F, Desbiens JF. Self-efficacy of physical and health education student teachers in the Quebec context. *Discourse Commun Sustain Educ.* 2021;12(1):22-41.

3. Jawaid M. Busy clinicians should develop a reading habit and learn time management: Dr. Masood Jawaid. *Pulse Int.* 2021;22(13):1-7.

4. Bonnstetter B, Suiter J. *The Universal Language of DISC Reference Manual.* Target Training International; 1984.

5. Qureshi FM, Bari SF, Siddiqui HJ, Tahir M, Khalid K, Rizwan S. Evaluation of patient satisfaction level with different outpatient department services: A situational analysis in a tertiary care hospital. *Pak Armed Forces Med J.* 2022;72(2):695-699.

6. Harding KE, Taylor NF. Highly satisfied or eager to please? Assessing satisfaction among allied health outpatients, including commentary by Haertl K. *Int J Ther Rehabil.* 2010;17(7):353-359. doi:10.12968/ijtr.2010.17.7.48892.

7. Badke MB, Sherry J, Sherry M, et al. Physical therapy direct patient access versus physician patient-referred episodes of care: Comparisons of cost, resource utilization & outcomes. *HPA Resour.* 2014;14(3):J1-J13.

8. Cheng, TZ, Gottfried ON, Dickson W, Park, C, Zakare-Fagbamila, R. The true penalty of the waiting room: The role of wait time in patient satisfaction in a busy spine practice. *J Neurosurg Spine.* 2020;33:95-105.

9. de Gruchy A, Granger C, Gorelik A. Physical therapists as primary practitioners in the emergency department: Six-month prospective practice analysis. *Phys Ther.* 2015;95(9):1207-1216. doi:10.2522/ptj.20130552.

10. Lentz TA, Goode AP, Thigpen CA, George SZ. Value-based care for musculoskeletal pain: Are physical therapists ready to deliver? *Phys Ther.* 2020;100(4):621-632. doi:10.1093/ptj/pzz171.

11. Hayhurst C. Good Fit: Physical therapy and value-based care. *APTA Mag.* 2022;14(5):42-50.

PART

3

PUTTING IT TOGETHER

This section provides guidance on mentorship and combines the individual concepts of professionalism to create a professional development plan for life-long growth

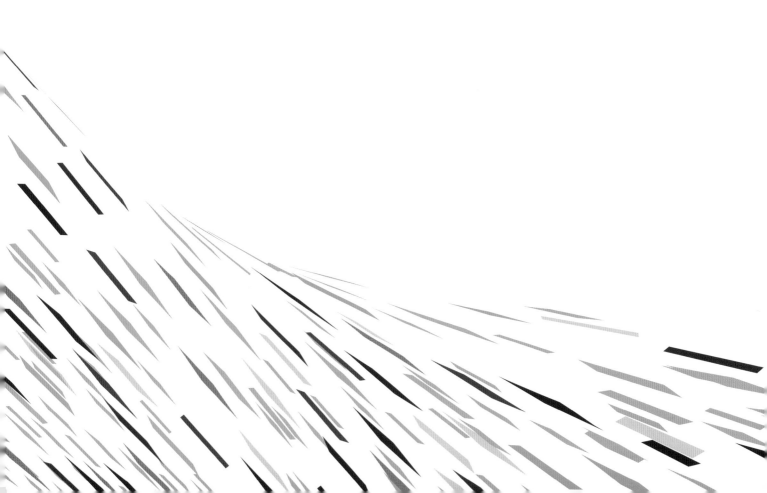

11

Mentorship and Professional Development

Now that we have explored professionalism and how it has evolved in medicine and physical therapy, it is time to focus on the role others play in helping us develop our professionalism. In this chapter, we explore the role of mentorship in professional development, formal assessment in mentorship, and mentorship in health care. Similar to the term professionalism, mentorship originated in ancient times. The term mentor comes from the Greek poem *Odyssey*. In Odyssey, the Goddess Athena took on the image of an older man, "Mentor," to guide young Telemachus to conquer his fears and enemies and help his father regain the throne.[1] These ancient origins still influence ideas of mentorship in the modern day. We often think of a mentor as an older, wiser individual who guides a younger person in their career and life quests. However, modern-day mentorship takes on a more complex concept than its ancient Greek origins. Today mentorship occurs in a variety of ways and relationships. For example, peers may mentor each other; individuals may participate in group mentorship programs, or you may consider cross-generational mentorship as a way to develop skills in different generations.[1-4] As we explore mentorship in this chapter, it is essential to have a working definition and a framework for building a productive mentoring relationship with others.

The social theory of social constructivism states that people learn from social experience and collaboration with others. Social constructivism provides a foundation for mentorship. Mentorship is a learning relationship in which the mentor and mentee collaborate to achieve goals, often professional development, for the mentee. The mentee grows personally and professionally through the connection to build knowledge and skills. Learning in mentorship occurs through scaffolding. Scaffolding refers to creating a supportive framework around the mentee and gradually removing the frame as the mentee gains independence in knowledge and skills. The mentor supports the mentee in learning and skill acquisition and may also champion the mentee's professional development by creating opportunities and facilitating network development. The mentoring relationship may be either an informal or formal relationship. Mentors and mentees need to understand the relationship and its expectations.[5-7] Let's explore the role of informal and formal mentorship in professional development.

● INFORMAL MENTORSHIP

There are no structured, planned interactions when mentoring is informal, and the mentor may be unaware they are acting as a mentor. Peer mentoring often occurs in this fashion. For example, someone begins a new position in an organization and connects to a coworker. Because of the level of comfort with the coworker, the new employee, the mentee, may choose to go to this person for guidance and support to gain organizational knowledge and skills and even to build their network. In this situation, the mentee and the mentor form an informal, well-defined mentorship with no real expectations. Although these relationships often occur in workplaces and serve a valuable purpose, they sometimes may cause resentment and frustration for both the mentor and mentee. Informal mentorships have no expectations established. Therefore, time commitment and resource allocation are not clearly defined. The lack of clarity or understanding about how much time and effort each person is willing to give to the mentoring relationship may become problematic. This can be rectified by clearly communicating that mentoring is occurring and establishing broad guidelines regarding the time and resources each person is willing to commit.[3,7]

Reflection Moment

1. Who has been an informal mentor to you? What skills and knowledge did they share? Did they realize they were your mentor?
2. Looking back on your life, have you been an informal mentor to anyone? What skills and knowledge did you share? How did you feel about the relationship? Did you realize you were a mentor?

● FORMAL MENTORSHIP

When long-term and structured mentoring is necessary, you should establish formal mentorship. Formal mentorship consists of structured meetings, goals, and clear expectations about the relationship. There are four phases of the formal mentorship relationship. The following section discusses the four phases.

Phases of Formal Mentoring

Phase 1: Preparation – This stage is often overlooked but is important in developing a foundation for mentoring. In this stage, the mentor and mentee examine their willingness and ability to engage in mentorship. The two should discuss time commitments, mentoring goals, and how each prefers to communicate. The use of formal assessment tools by the mentee can guide the mentoring process and is an important action in this phase. The following section discusses 360 evaluations and other useful formal assessments in mentorship. Another helpful step in this phase is for the mentee to clearly state their mentoring needs and ways they wish to participate. A document like "Me on a Page," outlined in **Table 11.1**, is useful in this mentorship phase.[1,6,8]

Phase 2: Negotiation – In this mentorship stage, the mentor and mentee develop the contract and set the foundation for the relationship. One of the biggest challenges in this stage this that individuals make assumptions about the relationship. It is vital to set clear expectations for both individuals and have a written agreement of those expectations. **Figure 11.1** is a sample contract that outlines goals, the structure of meetings, and the time commitment for mentorship. By having a contract, both parties understand their roles and mentorship.[1,6,8]

Phase 3: Enabling – The enabling phase is often what individuals think of when they envision mentorship. This stage is the active interaction between the mentor and the mentee. Important skills in this phase are communication skills, emotional intelligence, accountability, and self-management skills such as effective time use. It's important to reflect on documents completed during the preparation phase to ensure that mentoring stays focused and that each person is leveraging the most effective communication strategies and learning skills. During the enabling phase, the mentor uses scaffolding to support new skills and knowledge acquisition. As the mentee gains skills and knowledge, the mentorship moves into the feedback stage of mentoring.[1,6,8]

Phase 4: Feedback – Mentorship often moves back and forth between enabling and feedback. Mentors should provide both summative and formative feedback. Formative feedback occurs during the scaffolding in which the mentor provides guidance and insight during the course of learning to facilitate ongoing learning. In comparison, summative feedback is a more formal assessment. In summative feedback, the mentee and mentor review goals and objectives. They may revisit formal assessments such as a resilience scale or a cultural competency index to assess growth better. The mentor must understand how the mentee learns best and how they receive feedback to determine the best time and methods to provide mentoring feedback. Effective feedback is a powerful aspect of successful mentoring.[1,2,8]

Understanding the phases of formal mentorship and ensuring that mentorship moves through this phase is a way to establish a trusting and productive mentoring relationship. **Table 11.2** summarizes key concepts for each mentoring phase.

We discussed the specific tasks needed in each phase of mentoring. Both the mentor and mentee have particular responsibilities in mentorship. **Table 11.3** summarizes the mentor and mentee's responsibilities in formal mentorship.

1: We have agreed on the following goals and plan:	
Goals	Plan

2: We have discussed the following protocols by which we will work together:

Meeting times	
Communication methods	
Preparation for meetings	
Confidentiality	
Frequency and type of feedback	

We will meet regularly until we have accomplished our predefined goals for a maximum of ___ months. At the end of this time, we will review the agreement, evaluate our progress, and reach a learning conclusion. If we choose to continue our mentoring partnership, we will renegotiate this agreement.
Signed by both parties:

FIGURE 11.1. The Mentoring Contract.

TABLE 11.1. Me on a Page			
List Three Descriptions for Each Area			
How I like to Communicate			
How I Learn Best			
Ways I am Motivated			
What I Mommit to Bringing to My Mentoring			
Skills I Want to Develop			

TABLE 11.2.	Stages of Mentoring
Stages	**Steps to Take**
Preparation	Clearly define the time commitment. Examine goals for the interaction. Determine opportunities and barriers to communication. Take formal assessments to drive the interaction. Provide "Me on a Page."
Negotiation	Develop a work plan based on mentor, and mentee goals. Determine mentoring boundaries such as: frequency, materials shared, preparation expectations, confidentiality.
Enabling	Establish an open and affirming relationship. Monitor learning goals and work to keep focus and make progress. Ask open-ended questions that facilitate learning. Use active listening skills.
Feedback	Provide formative and summative content in a manner congruent with the mentee's communication and learning preference.

● REFLECTING ON MENTORING

As we discussed throughout this book, the act of reflection is a valuable tool for professional growth. In mentorship, reflection is a helpful tool for both the mentee and the mentor. Through ongoing reflection from session to session, the mentee and mentor can learn and grow professionally from the mentoring relationship. You may choose to use either informal or formal reflection. Informal reflection allows the person to review and clarify their thoughts throughout the process. In contrast, formal reflection guides the mentee and mentor in exploring specific topics. In the negotiation phase of mentoring, the individuals must establish expectations on sharing reflections. **Table 11.4** outlines some topics to consider for formal mentorship reflections.

TABLE 11.3.	Responsibilities of the Mentor and Mentee	
Mentor	**Mentee**	
Contract for the mentoring relationship Attendance and time management		
Manage each session	Prepare for the session	
Ensure the quality of each session	Establish learning needs	
Monitor the effectiveness of the relationship	Apply learning from the sessions	
Give feedback	Receive feedback	
Monitor ethical and professional issues	Expand self-awareness	
Keep notes Reflect and evaluate the process		

Adapted from Shaw[1]

TABLE 11.4.	Reflection on Mentoring
Reflecting	**Things to Consider**
At the End of Each Mentoring Session	1. What went well during the session? 2. What follow-up actions do I need to take? 3. What learning did we identify? 4. What was the quality of the communication and the interaction? 5. How could I work to improve the mentoring relationship?
Periodically Throughout the Mentoring Relationship	1. What is working in the mentoring partnership? 2. What could improve? 3. What key things am I learning through mentoring? 4. How are the learning goals being met? 5. What are my successes so far?

Formal mentorship incorporates the formation of goals and measurable objectives to assess the results of the mentee's growth through mentorship. As mentioned above, formal assessments are helpful in formal mentorship. Throughout this book, we discussed formal assessments as a measure of the different components of professionalism. Throughout your career, you may have the opportunity to participate in various formal assessment opportunities. These opportunities provide valuable insight into your professional development and help you to set professional goals. The following section briefly outlines a few of the assessments mentioned throughout this book and discusses other feedback tools.

Reflection Moment

Consider your educational and professional journey.

1. Have you participated in formal mentorship? If so, as a mentor, mentee, or both?
2. Did your mentorship experience include the four phases? Were any of the phases missed or incomplete? If so, how did that impact the mentorship experience?
3. Describe any assessment tools you used in formal mentorship. How did the formal assessment tools enhance the mentorship?

● FORMAL ASSESSMENTS

Feedback is a phase in the formal mentoring process; however, as professionals, we may receive feedback from others who are not acting as mentors. This feedback may come from a comment or remark made by a peer or a supervisor; it may come from a patient or client in the form of a satisfaction survey or a thank you note. Or it may come more formally, such as a performance review or a 360 evaluation. As professionals, reflecting on all types of feedback is essential in determining how best to integrate it into our professional growth. The formal feedback from performance reviews and 360 evaluations often offers constructive insight into our level of professional development and provides content for professional action plans and goal setting. Let's take a few minutes to discuss performance reviews and 360 evaluations.

You may be familiar with performance reviews, which is a review that usually occurs on an annual basis and provides a summary of an individual's performance as compared to an established standard, usually a job description. The performance review helps provide objective feedback regarding specific job duties and organizational expectations. This formal assessment often includes goals set in collaboration with a supervisor for continued job skill development. Although this type of assessment helps improve job skills, it often lacks insight into significant professional development, such as communication, emotional intelligence, and resilience.

The 360 evaluation, compared to the performance review, gives individuals insight into crucial professional development skills. This evaluation collects information regarding an individual's strengths and weaknesses from those around them. For example, a 360 evaluation might include information from supervisors, executive management, peers, direct reports, and patients/clients. The anonymous feedback from a 360 evaluation gives a comprehensive overview of an individual's ability to engage at all levels of an organization effectively. The 360 evaluation is a valuable tool for formal mentorship and compliments data from performance reviews and other standardized assessments, some of which were discussed in previous chapters, such as those listed in **Table 11.5**.

TABLE 11.5. Standardized Assessments in Mentoring	
Assessment	**Application to Mentoring**
DISC	Identifies your unique social and behavioral style and gives a framework for more effective communication in mentoring.
Emotional Quotient Inventory (EQ-i)	Provides an understanding of emotional intelligence. This tool gives information for goal setting and skill application to improve emotional intelligence.
Grit Scale (Grit-O)	The grit scale provides an understanding of two components of grit: passion and perseverance. This knowledge can help drive mentoring conversations around goals and focus.
Dweck Mindset Instrument	The Dweck Mindset Instrument provides an understanding of your fixed or growth mindset level. This instrument offers a foundation for discussion around achieving goals and skills acquisition.
Brief Resilience Scale	This scale measures your ability to bounce back from stressful events. This can allow you and your mentor to plan for stressful times in your life or career and gain new ways to manage stress.
Cross-Cultural Competency Inventory	This assessment provides an overview of cultural knowledge, emotion, and behaviors. This assessment can help plan and set goals for growth in cultural competency.

MENTORSHIP IN HEALTH CARE

As we discussed, mentoring occurs in many different ways. In health care, we see examples of other mentoring methods used to guide professional development. Let's review ways mentorship happens in health care.

Peer-to-Peer Mentorship

In the health care setting, peer-to-peer mentorship is a common occurrence. We mentioned the peer-to-peer mentorship that commonly occurs when someone is new to a role and connects to a peer in the same or similar role as an informal guide. Although this can be effective and helpful, this form of mentorship can cause challenges if time and resources are stretched for the mentor. In many health care organizations, formal peer-to-peer mentorship occurs. In this model, the mentor is often called a clinical instructor or a preceptor. The role of the formal peer mentor is to guide a student or a new employee in developing the skills and knowledge necessary to perform the role's duties effectively. In this model, preceptors or clinical instructors usually have additional training in mentoring techniques, and formal processes, assessments, and expected outcomes are established for the mentorship. This form of mentorship is an effective method in health care where the job roles of specific disciplines typically vary from setting to setting. For example, consider the role of a physical therapist in a hospital, outpatient clinic, or home health setting. Although foundational knowledge applies in each location, patient engagement roles, responsibilities, and specifics vary significantly. Even experienced clinicians find themselves requiring mentorship when changing health care settings.

Group Mentorship

The benefit of group mentoring is that group members learn from their mentors and peer mentees in the program. Limited time and resources in health care pose a threat to individual mentorship. Utilizing group mentorship improves efficiency and creates an environment for peer networking and relationship development that may otherwise not exist. Research on group mentoring for student clinicians found that participants

> **Programs for post-professional residency and fellowships exist in many health care professions, including physical therapy. The physical therapy residency programs have grown over the past few decades and now number more than 350 programs nationwide, according to the American Board of Physical Therapy Residency and Fellowship Education (ABPTRFE). Residency and fellowship programs include formalized mentorship, with an average of three to four hours of mentoring occurring weekly during the program for over twelve to fourteen months. The ABPTRFE provides accreditation for programs and standards for program content and structure.**

gained respect for each other's roles and improved their confidence, decision-making, and communication skills.[1]

Interdisciplinary Mentorship

When considering mentorship, we often think of a mentor who works in the same field as the mentee. However, there is significant value in participating in interdisciplinary mentorship. In the health care industry, interdisciplinary teams work together to provide patient care and lead organizations. Most clinicians will interact with members of other disciplines throughout their careers and may find themselves reporting to supervising team members from another field. Participating in mentorship with other disciplines provides opportunities to explore clinical care and leadership from a different perspective. It also allows team members to explore professional standards and guidelines from the perspective of other team members. As discussed in Chapter 10, networking is an important aspect of self-management. Interdisciplinary mentorship can lead to expanded networks for opportunities for growth in professional self-management.

Reflection Moment

Consider your educational and professional journey.

1. Describe the types of mentorship you experienced in your education or professional development.
2. List the positive and challenging aspects of each type of mentorship.

● A NOTE ON COACHING

The terms coach and mentor are often used interchangeably. However, differences exist between the two. As a professional, there may be times when you seek out a coach for a specific area of professional development. Unlike a mentor, a coach is often a paid individual whom a professional may employ to gain a deeper understanding of professional goals and challenges. Although both mentors and coaches may utilize similar techniques, the coach often has specialized training or certification related to coaching and may work in a different professional space than the person seeking coaching. Specific coaching areas include academic, leadership, business, and life coaching. Both mentors and coaches play a substantial role in professional development. Before seeking formal mentoring or coaching, understand your goals and the support a mentor or coach can provide toward achieving them.

● SUMMARY

This chapter defines mentorship and describes the many ways mentorship exists. This chapter provides insight into how you can seek out mentorship to support your professional development. Mentorship in professional development should be considered throughout your career, especially as an emerging professional, when you take on new roles and responsibilities, or when changing health care settings. As you gain experience and expertise as a reflective and influencing professional, consider how you can offer your knowledge and skills by becoming a mentor.

● PROFESSIONAL DEVELOPMENT

Reflection Moment

Take a moment to reflect on the role of mentorship in your career and how it may play a role in your future. Consider emerging, reflecting, and influencing professional levels and complete **Table 11.6**. In what ways may you need mentorship at each of these professional levels, and how might you provide mentorship at each of these professional levels?

Now, refer to **Table 11.7** to complete your professional strategic development plan for mentorship. Remember, completing the plan in each chapter helps build your overall professional development strategic plan at the end of the book.

TABLE 11.6. Mentorship Throughout Your Career		
	Ways I Could Benefit from Mentorship	Ways in Which I Could Mentor Others
Emerging		
Reflective		
Influencing		

TABLE 11.7. Professional Development Plan for Coaching and Mentoring		
Mentorship Goals (No More Than 2-3)	Tactics to Accomplish My Mentorship Goals	The Measure of Success for My Mentorship Goals

References

1. Shaw M, Fulton J. *Mentorship in Healthcare.* 2nd ed. M&K Publishing; 2015.

2. Brady B, Sidhu B, Jennings M, et al. The feasibility of implementing a cultural mentoring program alongside pain management and physical rehabilitation for chronic musculoskeletal conditions: results of a controlled before-and-after pilot study. *BMC Musculoskelet Disord.* 2023;24(1):47. doi:10.1186/s12891-022-06122-x.

3. Ibrahim HM, Shafri NAM, Tai J. Identifying opportunities for peer-assisted learning in speech language therapy clinical education. *Mengen Pasti Peluang Untuk Pembelajaran Berbantukan Rakan Sebaya Dalam Pendidik Klin Ter Bhs Pertuturan. Malaysian Journal of Health Sciences.* 2023;21(1):65-73.

4. Frese E, Cavallo C, Hawthorne K, Kettenback G, Yemm B. Faculty and student perceptions of a physical therapy professional behavior mentoring program. *Internet J Allied Health Sci Pract.* Published online September 7, 2021. doi:10.46743/1540-580x/2015.1548.

5. Toh RQE, Koh KK, Lua JK, et al. The role of mentoring, supervision, coaching, teaching, and instruction on professional identity formation: a systematic scoping review. *BMC Med Educ.* 2022;22(1):531. doi:10.1186/s12909-022-03589-z.

6. Ong YT, Quek CWN, Pisupati A, et al. Mentoring future mentors in undergraduate medical education. *PloS One.* 2022;17(9):e0273358. doi:10.1371/journal.pone.0273358.

7. Mullen CA, Klimaitis CC. Defining mentoring: a literature review of issues, types, and applications. *Ann N Y Acad Sci.* 2021;1483(1):19-35. doi:10.1111/nyas.14176.

8. Feeney MK, Bozeman B. Toward a useful theory of mentoring. *Adm Soc.* 2007;39:719-739.

chapter 12

Professional Development Plan

As you moved through the chapters in this book, you considered goals, strategies, and plans for each area of professional development. Now it's time to reflect on these areas collectively to create your professional development plan. Before you read this chapter, take some time and review the notes you made in the professional development section at the end of each chapter. Then, reflect on your current developmental level in each area and consider the goals you wrote. If a specific goal stands out to you in each section, highlight that goal.

In this chapter, we explore the components of strategic planning as a model for professional development. At the end of this chapter, you can combine your work throughout this book into a professional development plan to guide your future.

● STRATEGIC PLANNING AS A PROFESSIONAL DEVELOPMENT TOOL

Organizations use strategic planning to answer three vital questions: (1) Where are we now? (2) Where are we going? and (3) How will we get there? The strategic planning process provides a space to reflect on current actions and examine if these actions aid in moving forward. Strategic planning builds on three foundations: purpose, values, and vision. These foundations provide the road map that guides the organization in answering the three strategic questions.

This same process is helpful in professional development. In professional development, you begin with understanding your purpose, exploring your values, and creating a vision for yourself. From there, you work to answer the three strategic questions by building goals for professional development, determining tactics to achieve those goals, and deciding how to measure each goal's success. You might be thinking that this is very similar to clinical practice. As professionals in physical therapy, we use strategic thinking to guide our clinical practice. For example, the client/patient management

model uses evaluation and diagnosis to answer where is the patient/client now; client/patient interviews, prognosis, and goal setting to answer where is the patient/client going; and, finally, interventional strategies to determine how the client/patient gets there. The strategic thinking skills you develop as a clinician are helpful in your professional development planning. In the following portions of this chapter, use your strategic thinking skills to construct the foundation for professional development and create your unique professional development plan.

● PURPOSE, VALUES, VISION

Before creating a professional development plan, you must understand yourself as a person and professional. Insight into your purpose, values, and vision guides your growth to understand yourself as a professional better.

Professional Purpose

As a result of reflection, you should be able to develop a professional purpose statement. Your professional purpose statement is a brief, usually one-sentence, articulation of what matters most to you as a professional. This statement tells the world why you are a physical therapy professional. Most importantly, it gives you a starting point for professional development. When setting goals or actions related to your professional development, you first should reflect on your purpose and ask, "How does this goal or action serve my professional purpose? You may want to rethink the goal or activity if it doesn't fit your purpose. In this way, your purpose statement is your foundation for all professional growth. Your purpose statement may evolve throughout your career while maintaining very similar features. Therefore, revisiting and revising your purpose statement periodically may be prudent.

The Elevator Speech

Practicing the elevator speech is a great way to think about your purpose and develop your professional statement. The elevator speech briefly describes who you are as a professional. Consider riding in an elevator with another person, going from the first floor to the fifth floor, and the other person says, "Tell me about yourself." You have just a few moments to describe yourself to that person accurately. This practice is a powerful way to explore your thoughts and what is most important to you. The elevator speech gives insight into your purpose, vision, and goals. It is a great starting point for building the foundations of your professional development.

Let's take a moment to reflect on areas that help you write your purpose statement. You can understand your professional purpose by looking at some key questions:

Reflection Moment

Answer the following questions and complete the practice exercise.

1. List five words that describe you as a professional.
2. What am I passionate about in my profession?
3. What impact do I desire to have within the profession of physical therapy?
4. If I had two minutes, how would I describe myself as a professional?

Practice exercise: With a friend, peer, or mentor, practice your elevator speech. Use a timer so you stay brief in your description. Once you make your speech, have the other person tell you what key items they heard you say about yourself. Do this several times until you discover the correct terms and statements to describe yourself and your purpose clearly. You are ready to write your purpose statement once you answer the reflection questions and perform the elevator speech activity.

Values

In this book, we discussed the APTA core values as a guiding document for the profession of physical therapy. The nine core values guide members of the physical therapy profession in determining best practices and professional decision-making. Although the APTA core values are important to the profession, each individual should understand their values and how they interact with those established by the professional organization. Let's further explore values and the role they play in professional development.[1,2]

As humans, we often value those things that meet our needs. For example, something of value may fulfill a biological need, such as food and water or, on a higher level, a social need, such as trust or honesty. We most often consider what values we hold in social connection. Values have specific attributes. These attributes give insight into the values' vital role in driving decisions and framing our lives. **Table 12.1** lists the attributes of values and provides examples of how they drive decisions and interactions with others.[3]

The attributes listed in Table 12.1 demonstrate the power of values and their role in our lives. As stated in the third attribute, values transcend situations. Therefore, our values in our personal lives reflect in our professional lives. Our values help to drive the decisions

---

Write Your Purpose Statement Here:

TABLE 12.1. Attributes of Values	
Attributes	**Examples**
1. Values are beliefs linked to affect. Activating values triggers feelings	When my values are threatened, I may feel anger. For example, if I value the trust and someone breaks it, I may feel angry toward them.
2. Values reflect a desired outcome and may motivate action.	Values drive your goals and actions. For example, I value altruism. Therefore, I may set a goal to give back to the community, and my action is volunteering for a community nonprofit.
3. Values transcend specific actions and situations	Your values do not change based on circumstances. For example, I may value trust. This value exists in my personal relationships and professional relationships.
4. Values serve as a standard or criteria for judging things as good or bad.	We often place our values as a judgment on circumstances and other humans. Although this can help with decision-making, it can be a blind spot and cause us to judge circumstances and others unfairly. For example, if I value the trust and someone breaks my trust in a situation, I may use that value to decide that person is bad. It's important that we stay aware of this attribute and evaluate our judgments of circumstances and others.
5. Values have an order of importance.	Some values have more meaning for us than others, and we may choose to sacrifice one value for another. For example, if I value achievement and security but value achievement more than security, I may sacrifice security for the next step toward achievement.

Adapted from Schwartz, 2012[3]

TABLE 12.2. Values Assessment Tools

Value Assessment Tool	Description
Schwartz Portrait Values Questionnaire (PVQ)	There are long and short versions of this assessment. This is one of the most universally accepted values assessments. Based on ten fundamental values which influence human action.
Personal Values Assessment (PVA)	Short and straightforward assessment which measures core values and personal beliefs. Classifies values into three sub-types: personal, social, and universal.
Valued Living Questionnaire (VLQ)	Determines values based on ten domains of living. It examines how individuals regard their values and incorporate them into actions.

regarding our chosen profession, how we interact each day in our professional settings, and our career goals and aspirations.

There are many different ways we can explore our values. For example, we can reflect on circumstances and interactions with others and consider what values drove those decisions. There are formal assessments that help to determine our motivations and values. There are also lists of values available to rank and determine which values resonate with you. **Table 12.2** below lists three different reliable and valid values assessment tools.[4]

Whether you use a formal assessment tool or take time to reflect on and research values, it is crucial to articulate your values and understand how they influence your professional development. The reflection moment below gets you started in understanding your values.

Reflection Moment

Take 10-15 minutes to create a list of words that come to mind when you think about your values. Based on this list, write a brief sentence about why these values matter to you. Put the list aside and revisit it over the next few days. Allow some time for thought, and then take some time to rank them in the level of importance to you. Once you determine the order of your values, share the list with a close friend, peer, or mentor and discuss them in more detail. Repeat this practice until you feel comfortable with your values and their role in your life.

Vision Statement

Your vision statement is an extension of your purpose statement. The vision statement is designed to answer the question, "Where are you going?" It doesn't have an endpoint but provides the horizon to strive for in your career. Throughout this book, we discussed the APTA's vision statement, "Transforming society by optimizing movement to improve the human experience."[5] This doesn't have an endpoint. We can continue transforming society and improving movement and the human experience; this statement inspires professional growth. We can reflect on how our actions are moving the profession toward transforming society. Your vision statement should reflect this same type of aspiration. Perhaps you want to impact the lives of a specific group of individuals through your actions as a physical therapy professional, or maybe you want to guide national health policies or transform an aspect of the profession through your research endeavors. Your vision statement should reflect your specific passion for the profession of physical therapy, build on your strengths, and reflect your values. It should inspire you to act and move forward. Well-thought-out vision statements drive professional development goals and let you envision your professional road ahead.

Let's take a moment to reflect on your passions, strengths, and values and create your professional vision statement.

Reflection Moment

Consider the following questions:

1. What strengths do I bring to my profession?
2. What am I most passionate about in my profession?
3. What am I most passionate about in my personal life?
4. How do my passions and values connect?

Practice exercise: Envision that you have had a long and remarkable career, and now it's time to retire. A close colleague is speaking at your retirement celebration and has a few moments to summarize the impact of your career. Write the speech for your colleague. After writing this speech, compare the speech

Write a Brief and Powerful Statement of Your Professional Vision Here:

to your answers to the questions above. Use this information to create a brief and powerful statement of your professional vision.

● CREATING A PROFESSIONAL DEVELOPMENT PLAN

By this point in the book, you have done much work building the foundation for an effective professional development plan. You have determined goals, tactics, and strategies for each area of professionalism in chapters 4-10, and you have explored your purpose, values, and vision. Now, it is time to build a professional development plan to guide you in the next phase of your career.

At the beginning of this chapter, we discussed the three questions that strategic planning answers and how they connect to your professional development plan. **Figure 12.1** demonstrates the process for professional development planning. At the foundation are your purpose, values, and vision. From that foundation, you begin to explore where you are now. Are you an emerging, reflective, or influencing professional, and what areas are the most important to focus on moving toward the next level of professionalism? Once you establish these areas, use your vision to determine where you want to go and what specific goals will help you to get there. Finally, you put the plan in place. How are you going to get there? What are the necessary actions to achieve the goals, and how will you measure the success of those outcomes?

Now it's time to create your strategic development plan. Your plan should include your purpose, values, vision, professional development level, and three to five prioritized goals for your future development. When developing your priorities, each should include a goal, a tactic, a measure of success, and an accountability partner. The first component is the goal itself. Just like clinical goal setting, these goals should follow the SMART framework:

- *Specific*
- *Measurable*
- *Achievable*
- *Relevant*
- *Time-bound*

Next, the tactics should include specific actions that help you achieve the established goals. These tactics might be broad statements, but if so, they should break down into specific tangible small steps. For example, if a tactic is to read literature, you might break that down to one article monthly. Then, your measures of success should be a demonstration of achieving your goal. For example, suppose your goal is to obtain a specialization certification. In that case, a measure of success might be completing the exam in that specialty area or being recognized as a leader in your work environment. Finally, identifying an accountability partner helps set the stage for future success in achieving these goals. Telling someone or working collaboratively with someone to reach goals provides motivation and guidance in goal achievement. **Table 12.3** provides a framework for your professional development plan. Create 3-5 prioritized goals.

Putting Your Plan into Action

Congratulations! As you moved through this book, you have done much work exploring your professional journey.

- *You now have an understanding of yourself as an emerging, reflecting, or influencing professional*
- *You have examined your strengths and challenges in aspects of professionalism*
- *You have discovered your professional purpose, values, and mission*

Now it's time to put that plan into action! At this point in professional development, it's easy to put all this work aside, get caught up in our day-to-day activities, and wait to follow through on the plan. Unfortunately, it happens within organizations all the time; teams spend hours working through an analysis of the organization and developing a thorough strategic plan, only to put it aside and get caught up in daily work until it's time to revisit the plan in a year or so. So, let's ensure you have the strategies necessary to move your plan forward.

- **Write it down!** Add actions that move you toward your goals on a calendar or somewhere that will remind you to reflect on your goals.

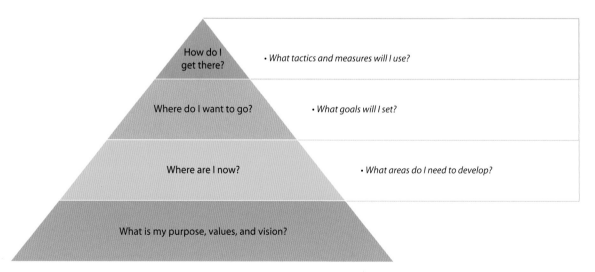

FIGURE 12.1. Process of Professional Development.

TABLE 12.3. Professional Development Plan			
My Purpose			
My Values			
My Vision			
My Current Professional Level (Emerging, Reflective, Influencing) (Describe why.)			
Professional Development Goal	Tactic to Achieve My Goal	Measure of Success	Accountability Partner for This Goal

- **Eat the elephant!** How do you eat an elephant? One bite at a time! Take on those goals one small piece at a time. Take each tactic, break it into smaller steps, and act on those small steps.

- **Be accountable!** In Chapter 7, we addressed accountability. Think of your goals in those statements that help you move forward toward actions. Don't get caught in the language that places barriers in your way. For example, "I need to wait to work on that goal until I have more time," or "My work is so busy right now it's hard to find time to read those articles." These thoughts will stand in your way.

- **Don't go it alone!** Remember that you placed accountability partners in each of your reflections on professional development and within the overall plan. Rely on these people to help nudge you along to success. Also, remember those mentors and coaches and their role in your professional development.

By using these strategies, you will set yourself up for success in your professional development.

● LIFELONG PROFESSIONAL DEVELOPMENT

Chapter 10 discussed lifelong learning and its essential role in our professional life. Professions evolve as their members continue to learn and grow and develop themselves. Our duty as physical therapy professionals is to continue this journey. We designed this book as a resource that can be referenced throughout your career. As you move from an emerging professional through a reflecting phase into an influencing professional,

revisit the chapters in this book and reflect on your professional development. Take the time to examine your purpose and vision and remind yourself of those values that drive your actions and decisions. Update your professional development plan every few years. Making this practice part of your journey will enrich your career and the lives of those you serve as a physical therapy professional.

References

1. Anderson D. *A Validation Study of the APTA Professionalism in Physical Therapy Core Values Self-Assessment.* Northern Illinois University; 2015.
2. Denton J, Fike DS, Walk M, Jackson C. Test-retest reliability of the APTA professionalism in physical therapy: core values self-assessment tool in DPT students. *J Phys Ther Educ Sect.* 2017;31(4): 2-7. doi:10.1097/JTE.0000000000000001.
3. Schwartz SH. An overview of the Schwartz theory of basic values. *Online Read Psychol Cult.* 2012;2. https://search.ebscohost.com/login.aspx?direct=true&AuthType=sso&db=edsair&AN=edsair.doi..........19119709c95d4fde85b7938c42ac96de&site=eds-live&scope=site&custid=s4786267.
4. Chowdhury M. The 3 best questionnaires for measuring values. *Positive Psychology.* Published August 12, 2019. https://positivepsychology.com/values-questionnaire/#:~:text=The%20Personal%20Values%20Assessment%20(PVA)%20is%20a%20short%20and%20straightforward,to%20our%20core%20personal%20values. Accessed March 25, 2023.
5. *APTA Vision, Mission, and Strategic Plan.* https://www.apta.org/apta-and-you/leadership-and-governance/vision-mission-and-strategic-plan.

Index

Note: Page numbers followed by *f* indicate figures; and page numbers followed by *t* indicate tables.